Surviving HIV

Growing Up a Secret and
Being Positive

JAMIE GENTILLE

Cover art by Cami Frickman
www.graygoosestudios.com

Author photo by Kerri Ellsworth

ISBN: 1482575930
ISBN-13: 9781482575934

For my family and friends

CHAPTER ONE

I was a sack of rice with a heart defect. If there isn't a country song out there with this title, there should be. *Sack of Rice with a Heart Defect...the saloon door's broke and so's my leaky valve.* Done. It's a sure hit. You're welcome, country music industry. In addition to being a musical hit, this is how I started out on this little journey of mine. We couldn't have known that my life wouldn't exactly be smooth sailing on the day I made my debut into this world. It was August. It was hot, I'm assuming; I was there, but I don't really remember the weather. My mom was in the grocery store when her labor pains started, which is very fitting because I love food, and I probably just wanted a snack. So I decided it was time to come out.

My mom, thinking she was just having back pains, continued her shopping, all hunched over her cart. Aisle by aisle, she slowed down a bit and hunched over a little more. Milk. Eggs. Fruit Roll-Ups.

Contraction. Cheerios. Oreos. Contraction. Wonder Bread. Contraction.

When she got home she decided that she needed to rest, so my dad took my sisters, Kelly and Heather, out to dinner to give my mom some peace and quiet. By the time they got home from dinner, her back pains were five minutes apart and she realized that they were actually contractions. Everyone piled into the car and headed to the hospital. My mom got settled in and my dad, a professional coffee drinker, headed to the cafeteria for a cup. By the time he got his coffee, stirred in his four sugars, and made it back to my mom, I had arrived. Clearly, I was in no mood for dilly-dallying. I was ten pounds of slimy baby. Ten pounds. This would explain why everyone thought that my mom was having twins. At one point during her pregnancy, the doctor thought he heard two heartbeats, when in reality it was just my own heartbeat echoing in the cavernous space that I was created in there. Ten pounds of pure newborn joy. I recently picked up a 10-pound bag of rice at Costco and I instantly called my mother to apologize. Carrying that bag of rice from the store to the car to my apartment was bad enough; I can't imagine lugging it around in my uterus 24 hours a day and then—oh God, this hurts to even think about—birthing it. Good God. I need to start giving my mom better Mother's Day gifts. And let's be honest: on my birthday, she should really get all the presents.

So my parents had their third in a series of adorable little girls. Kelly, Heather, and rice sack Jamie. I would love to be able to say that I was the cutest, but that just wasn't the case. I've seen the pictures, and it wasn't pretty. I looked like Winston Churchill if he were greased down and really mad. I was definitely the biggest though, so my sisters can't take that away from me. Two weeks later, my mom brought her mega baby in for my check-up. The receptionist probably thought one of two things. One: Man, that mom sure procrastinates. Why is she just now bringing her four-month old in for her two-week check-up? or two: Wow, what a cute and very large child-baby.

What was expected to be a normal check-up brought some unexpected news. The doctor heard an unusual sound on my heart exam. Babies have a blood vessel that functions in utero to divert blood from the lungs directly to the body, as the baby's lungs get all of its oxygenated blood through the mother's placenta. This vessel is not needed after birth, and it typically closes up on its own. Sometimes it doesn't close up right away, creating an extra heart sound. The doctor thought that this was the case with me, and told my mother that we should give it a month; it would probably close up on its own.

One month passed, and we went to check it out. Lo and behold, it was still there. I do things on my own time, but this was rather worrisome. The doctor recommended that we give it another month, which went over like a lead balloon with my mom. Relying on her dead-on maternal instincts and fierce protective sense, she demanded more testing. At the ripe old age of 2 months, I had my first electrocardiogram (EKG) to evaluate the electrical conductivity of my heart. It

3

showed nothing remarkable. With no definite answers, we went on with life.

"It's probably nothing," the doctor said. "If something is wrong with her heart, you will see warning signs before anything happens. Her lips will turn blue. Just keep an eye on her." Comforting. I was like my own personal mood ring. Pink = happy and healthy. Blue = hey, you should probably call 911. No big deal.

Months passed with my parents keeping their watchful eyes on me, and I seemed to be growing like a normal baby. No blue lips, no warning signs. Things were looking up. I was developing more and discovered an amazing new skill – crawling. It was such a milestone for me and for my parents, since they now had to keep up with a mobile baby who didn't just lie on her back like an overturned turtle. This is when the fun really began.

That summer, when I was 11 months old, we visited family friends, Sandy and Charlie, in Oklahoma. They lived on a farm with all sorts of animals—cows, horses, barn cats, barn kittens (my favorite), armadillos, and snapping turtles. Oklahoma: the petting zoo of Middle America. As a young child, I came to adore this place; all the kittens I could cuddle! A little girl's dream and a barn kitty's nightmare.

One afternoon, my mom was chatting with Sandy as I crawled around. I started crawling from my mom to Sandy, and something happened. My body went stiff as a board, and then I collapsed. Terrified, my mom scooped me up and drove me to the local hospital. A limp noodle in her arms, I did finally wake up in the car after a few terrifying moments. By the time we got to the hospital, I seemed relatively normal and the doctors, again, found nothing remarkable. They sent us home with the same prescription: to "keep an eye on her." Mom called my dad to tell him what had happened; thoroughly freaked out himself, he told my mom to call the doctor at home. She did, and he advised her not to rush home unless it happened again. We made it through the end of the trip with no other incidents, and made a bee-line for the doctor when we got home.

I had another EKG, which was again, unremarkable. The doctor began to think it was something related to my neurological functioning, so they did some neurological tests. Unremarkable. By this time, I'm sure I was quite tired of being called unremarkable. What a lackluster assessment. Couldn't they throw me a bone? "Well folks, Jamie's test was unremarkable, but we think that she herself is quite remarkable. Look at those eyes!" I'm just saying.

Alas, my unremarkable brain worked just fine, so they explored other options. I have been a strong-willed little person since I was born, so the doctor suggested that maybe I was holding my breath and passing out to get attention. I would have been one very calculating and manipulative one-year-old if this were the case. I'm stubborn, but not that stubborn. If this were truly the case, I would have my own reality show by now. It would be called The Remarkable Baby. My parents knew that wasn't it, and that there was something there that everyone was missing.

Meanwhile, my spells began occurring more frequently. I would pass out cold—not a fun party trick at all, and one that scared the bejesus out of my family and anyone around me. My parents began to notice that these spells occurred when I was more active, so to prevent them from happening, they tried to keep me as inactive as possible. Have fun with that one, oh parents of a one-year-old. Any parent knows that it's nearly impossible to keep a growing baby still, but there is usually one magical place where that happens: the car seat. Thus, my mom put me in the car and we drove around and around so that I would just zone out. Zone-out therapy did work, but my parents knew there was something seriously wrong with me and we had to figure it out, because this just wasn't a long-term solution. The gas prices alone would do us in.

Throughout these fainting episodes, my mom thought, What am I NOT saying to these doctors to get them to take this seriously? She described my episodes, but I had yet to have active symptoms in the presence of a doctor. At times, my mom worried that they thought she was exaggerating everything for attention. This process was heartbreaking and frustrating for my parents, but they didn't let up.

At the doctor's office one day, my mom asked the doctor, "How much do you trust a mother's instinct?"

He said, "Yours, I would trust."

"I know it's her heart. We have to do more testing to see what's going on with her heart."

The doctor reluctantly agreed to schedule a heart catheterization for the following week. This is an invasive procedure used to diagnose certain heart conditions; a catheter is threaded into the heart through the groin or neck. It's no walk in the park for a one-year-old, but the doctor trusted my mom's instincts and scheduled the test.

The Thursday prior to my heart catheterization, I had my worst spell yet. I was with my sisters in the living room, and I collapsed. Kelly screamed at the top of her lungs for my mom, and she came running in, knowing what must have happened. My mom picked up her lifeless one-year-old and raced to the hospital. I woke up and was back to my normal self by the time we got to the hospital, but my mom demanded that I be admitted until we had the heart catheterization. She didn't think I was going to make it through the weekend.

There, we began our first of many hospital stays. The staff were skeptical of why I was staying at the hospital before my procedure, because I looked like a normal, healthy toddler. When the doctors did their morning rounds, they said, "This patient is admitted because her mom is worried about her," and it was obvious to my mom that no one took her seriously. At this point, though, she didn't care. I was in the hospital, the safest place I could be when my next spell happened.

During our pre-procedure stay, my mom took me all over the hospital in my stroller—the gift shop, the cafeteria—anywhere to break up the monotony of the day and to keep me from exerting myself. She got to know other patients and even cuddled them when their parents weren't there. This was before the days of patient confidentiality, and she became the mama bear of the unit. This is my mom to a T: always taking care of the little ones around her.

Waiting. Strolling. Playing. Passing the time.

Then the most miraculous and terrifying thing happened. The nurses were gathered for their shift change, giving reports on their patients. I was with my mom in the orange, carpeted hallway pushing a baby doll stroller. Just like any other afternoon there, the two of us together, getting through the day. And it happened again. I tensed up, went limp as a noodle, and then collapsed. My mom scooped me up in her arms and ran to the room where the nurses were giving report. The door was closed, and my mom kicked it in, action-hero-style, and yelled, "She's doing it again!" The nurses were shocked that I was lifeless in my mom's arms, and that this crazy mom wasn't so crazy after all. They saw it with their own eyes, and from that point forward, they all took my mom seriously. It was a blessing in disguise; finally, other people were there to witness that this was in fact really happening.

From that point forward, I wasn't allowed to leave the nursing unit, and I was strictly monitored. No one knew when I would collapse again, and if the next spell would kill me. We made it through the weekend and I finally had my heart catheterization. This was the first time that a diagnostic test actually revealed something remarkable — incredibly remarkable, as it turned out.

I had a condition called Tetrology of Fallot, a very serious congenital heart defect that affects the flow of blood through the heart. This condition consists of four major defects of the heart: ventricular septal defect (VSD), pulmonary stenosis, right ventricular hypertrophy, and an overriding aorta. A VSD is a hole between the left and right ventricles that allows oxygen-rich and oxygen-poor blood to mix together. Pulmonary stenosis is a narrowing of the pulmonary valve, which allows blood to go into the pulmonary artery to the lungs to pick up oxygen. Right ventricular hypertrophy is a thickening of the ventricle wall that results from the heart working harder to push blood through the narrowed pulmonary valve. An overriding aorta means that the main artery that brings oxygenated blood to the body is picking up oxygen-poor blood in the mix. All of these defects result in the body not receiving enough oxygenated blood. Basically, my little heart was a hot mess.

The doctors were astonished to see how damaged my heart was. They were even more astounded that I was still alive, considering how severe my condition was. This is where my stubbornness comes in; I defied the laws of medicine that said that I should have already died by the time I was a year old. Lucky for me, I'm not much of a rule-follower.

CHAPTER TWO

IN my first 12 months of life, I had accumulated a thicker medical file than most adults. While the average parent worried about thumb sucking and potty training, mine worried about finding the right diagnostic test, and the threat of their baby dying in their arms. Kelly, ten years older than me, and Heather, four years older than me, were getting used to having a little sister who was very fragile and required a lot of attention. I was like their pet bonsai tree.

Although my diagnosis was grave, it was at least something tangible. We finally had answers—terrifying ones, but answers nonetheless. With a definitive diagnosis in hand, it was time to move on with a plan. My messed up little heart could not be mended with medications, and we certainly couldn't go on with me becoming cyanotic anytime I decided to move. I was like a hairdryer that cut out after it ran too long. A victim of faulty wiring! And that's no fun for anyone, really.   Surgical intervention was the only option.

There were several options on the surgical menu. The doctors discussed replacing my crappy leaky valves with artificial valves; this would certainly fix the problem, but it also meant a lifetime of surgically upgrading valves as I grew. It's hard enough to keep up with a kid's growing shoe size, much less a cardiac valve, so that was not the best option for me. Another option was a Blalock-Taussig shunt procedure. This procedure is meant as a temporary solution to treat Tetrology of Fallot; here, the subclavian artery is redirected to the pulmonary artery to allow more blood to flow to the lungs for oxygenation. Imagine you're on the highway (right ventricle) and all of a sudden it narrows to one measly lane (defected pulmonary valve). You're not going anywhere, and you really need to get to this party – the Get Oxygenated in the Lungs (G.O.L) Party. Then, a road crew (the brilliant surgeon) builds a bigger, wider road (shunt) that you can hop onto to get to your G.O.L. party.   That's your basic shunt procedure, and it tides you over until you can get the more aggressive surgery. Like a snack before dinner.

The third surgical option was the whole shebang. Go in there with guns blazing and fix everything at once with the mack daddy procedure. The advantage was that it theoretically fixes the entire four-tiered problem. One and done. The downside: it was an incredibly invasive surgery for a one-year-old, and it takes a huge toll on such young and fragile patients. The surgeons would widen or replace the pulmonary valve and patch up the VSD. Sounds simple enough, but it's invasive and the cardiovascular surgeons had never performed this procedure on anyone as young as 12 months before. This was certainly not an area in which my parents wanted me to be the first. They opted for the snack – a Blalock shunt to tide me over until I was strong enough to have the big whopper surgery.

At 14 months old, I was scheduled to have my shunt surgery. The plan was to reroute a large artery (the one that went to my right arm) to my pulmonary artery. It was a terrifying time for my family, yet it was the first time we were moving in the right direction. Going into the procedure, the doctor told my parents that I would likely have some paralysis on my right side, which may or may not resolve itself—there would be no way to predict whether it would be permanent. An invasive heart procedure wasn't enough; we had to throw some unpredictable paralysis into the mix.

It was go time, and we were ready for this monumental step. After the procedure, the waiting game began. Sure enough, I woke up with facial paralysis. The right side of my face drooped, and my right eye didn't open. Only time would tell if this would return to normal. At this point, my dad made a pact with whatever higher power was listening and vowed that if my right eye opened, he would quit smoking. This higher power was clearly a non-smoker, because sure enough, after a few days – hello starshine! – my eye opened. The paralysis resolved itself, and I made a full recovery. And Dad stopped smoking.

The surgery was a roaring success, and my heart now had a specially made route for oxygenating my blood. I could now be a normal toddler, playing and exploring my world without becoming cyanotic. And honestly, the world is a much better place when you're conscious. Ask anyone who's had a bad night in Vegas and they'll back me up on that one.

The success of the procedure carried me through the next year and a half. These were also very formative months of toddler development and I became more aware of my environment. I continued to be a frequent flyer at the hospital, always coming back for check-ups, echocardiograms (echoes), and EKGs to ensure that the little ticker was still holding on strong.

When we drove into the dark garage of the hospital, I knew exactly where we were. As we got out of the car, I clung to my mom a little tighter because I knew that being at the hospital meant I would get poked and prodded. The environment around us was frenzied, and smelled like gasoline. The world got bigger and I got smaller when I came to the hospital.

We walked into the building through the automatic sliding doors from the garage. The entrance to the hospital had ascending and descending moving walkways that seemed to go on forever. It was one of the fun parts of my visits – like an Epcot Center ride – really slow, but really fun! It got less and less fun however, as we reached the top level. Another set of sliding doors brought us into the open atrium of the hospital lobby. It felt like being in a museum, filled with dozens of people in a big, bright, open space.

Everyone seemed busy. A constant low roar of activity buzzed around us as we walked to the registration area.

My anxiety was always alleviated when I saw the bright orange and yellow bucket chairs. These were the coolest things ever made. They looked like they belonged in the Jetson's living room: shiny, sleek little pods that spun around if you pushed with your feet. They were like giant M&Ms with a spot to sit. I made myself dizzy on these things while my mom checked me in at registration. Thank God I'd had the shunt surgery before I was old enough to go crazy on those chairs, because the dizziness would not have helped my daily plight of staying conscious.

I played on the bucket chairs while we waited to go back for my appointment, which usually consisted of blood work, an echo, and an EKG. My excitement with the chairs was always tempered with anxiety because I knew that at any moment we would have to go back for my appointment. It had been months since my shunt surgery, and my appointments were usually pretty quick, but I always had a fear that when they took me back, they would do surgery on me again. It lingered in the back of my head the whole time we were there, during every appointment.

When the nurse called my name, I stopped spinning and looked at my mom as if to say, Do we really have to go back with her? She comforted me and told me exactly what we were going to do so there wouldn't be any unpleasant surprises. I got up willingly and followed the nurse with my mom. The hallways were carpeted—back in the days when they put carpet in hospitals—with lovely earth tones of burnt sienna, Dijon mustard yellow, and brick red. The wall décor conveniently accented these rich tones, creating a veritable autumn-hued nightmare. God bless the 70s.

Our first stop was the lab, to get my blood drawn. We sat in a smaller waiting room that was much less fun; the walls were white and there was usually one sad-looking toy in the corner. There wasn't much to do here but think about getting stuck with the needle. At this point, I sat on my mom's lap, just hoping they would forget about me or run out of needles. No such luck. They called my name and we went back.

I sat on my mom's lap while the lab technician got all the tubes and supplies lined up. When the technician put on her gloves, I buckled down for the poke. I never struggled or fought, because I knew it wouldn't get me anywhere. Luckily, my mom was great at hugging me tight and telling me that I was doing a great job. I watched the technician as she tied the tourniquet around my bicep and cleaned off my arm with alcohol. That antiseptic smell made me tense up, knowing that seconds later would be the needle. I never looked away, because I needed to see everything that was happening. As the needle went in, I usually whimpered in pain, but kept watching. My arm became numb and purple from the tourniquet, and I watched as she drew tube after tube of blood. Finally, she released the tourniquet, and I got feeling back in my arm. When the needle came out, I felt my favorite emotion on the planet: relief. The tough part was over and I could finally relax.

The next part of my appointment was at the cardiology clinic, where we checked in and waited in yet another waiting room. This one wasn't nearly as daunting, because I wasn't worried about my labs anymore. The next test on our list was the EKG. We walked back to the exam room for what my mom and I called the 'kisser test.' The EKG machine consisted of several suction cups, all connected to a central machine with small wires. The suction cups were small rubber bulbs affixed to a metal cup. They resembled tiny bike horns, and they made "kissing" sounds when they were removed.

I laid down on the table and the tech squirted goop (gel) on several different spots on my chest, arms, and ankles. On each blob of goop, she attached one "kisser" by squeezing the bulb and suctioning it onto my skin. I looked like one of Frankenstein's projects, but it was painless. I lay still for a few minutes and the test was done. Next was the fun part; as each kisser came off, it made a SCHLURRRRP sound, which always made me laugh. Un-schlurped, I wiped off all of the goop and went to the next room for my echo.

This test was not as much fun. For this one, I lay down on the table and got all gooped up again. Instead of kissers, though, the tech put stickers on my chest. Really sticky stickers. I hated that part, because I knew those stupid stickers would eventually have to come off, and that was no fun. I lay down and the tech put the transducer on my chest to start the exam. It was about the size of a computer mouse, and apart from sometimes pushing hard into my ribs, it was painless.

For some reason, though, I was always a little worried that something like a needle would shoot out of it, into my skin. This is where my toddler imagination came in. So I lay there perfectly still, waiting quietly for it to be over. The room was dark so the tech could see the screen, which showed a blurry image of my beating heart. It was always interesting to watch, even though I had no idea what I was looking at. After about 15 minutes the test was over, and the tech would always happily say, "We're all done!" Oh yeah, lady, I thought, then why are these stickers still all over me? I know we're not done yet.

This part sucked.

The tech started to pull off the stickers and my tears started flowing. At this point, my mom always jumped in to ask if she could pull them off. This was a relief, because I knew she would be as gentle as possible. After they were off, I felt my favorite feeling of relief again.

Our last stop of the day was to see my cardiologist, Dr. Perry. I sat on the paper-covered table with my mom, waiting for him to come in. He opened the door with a big smile, always happy to see me. He walked over to me and gave my nose a honk. He listened to my heart and lungs, making me giggle the whole time. I never felt scared with Dr. Perry, because he was just a funny guy in a white coat.

When we were done in Dr. Perry's office, we headed back to the big atrium for my favorite stop of the day – the gift shop. I could rattle off the entire inventory of that place after all the times we visited it. Throughout all those painful procedures and pokes, I was always comforted by the fact that my day would end at the gift shop. I picked out my treasure for the day, and off we went.

Months passed, and I continued to grow as an active toddler. My second surgery was scheduled when I turned 2, but I was doing so well after my shunt surgery that it was decided I could hold off even longer for the big shebang. The older and stronger I got, the greater chance I had of making it through such invasive surgery. I was a growing and thriving toddler, experiencing the normal joys of being a kid.

As a family, we spent hours in our pool, swimming away the hot summer days. My parents taught us how to swim practically before we could walk, and I presented an even greater challenge for them on that front. Most people can recall a staple of American childhood – the floatie. These inflatable donuts wrap kids' biceps and effectively kept them afloat while they learn to swim. Swimmers' training wheels. It was time for me to make that rite of passage, so my mom took me out to our pool, slathered me with sunblock, and took out the floaties. I looked at them in absolute horror. What sort of barbaric devices of torture where those?? When I realized that she actually wanted to put these inflatable donuts from hell ON MY ARMS, I lost my head. I screamed and kicked, as if she was trying to tie barbed wire around my spindly little arms. The poor neighbors probably called Child Protective Services and Animal Control that day.

I wanted absolutely nothing to do with those horrible

things. Up to that point in my life, the only things wrapped around my arms like that were blood pressure cuffs and tourniquets that squeezed the living daylights out of me. That feeling of something on my arm meant being in the hospital, being uncomfortable, and being afraid. Any remote suggestion of that in my normal life made me panic, so floaties and I were not friends.

My mom, being the intuitive and all-knowing mom that she is, knew exactly why I freaked out like a rabid raccoon. She also knew that she would have to figure out another way to help me learn how to swim. In search of a Plan B, we went to Toys R Us. To me, it was just another fun trip to the toy store, but my mom was on a covert mission; she knew she would have to be stealthy with any attempt to get me to like a flotation device. I sat in the cart as we rolled through the aisles full of treasures. We made stops at my favorite sections: the bike aisle, where I could test-drive the miniature cars; the huge vat of balls I would bounce across the aisle; and my all-time favorite, the Cabbage Patch doll section. I was in heaven.

When we rolled into the summertime swim section, I was engrossed in the wonderment of all the pool toys, and my mom started looking for an alternative flotation device. She found a floatie that tied around the waist instead of the arms. Perfect. She quietly placed it in the back of the cart, as gingerly as if it were a soufflé with a bomb in it. Hoping that we could get out of the store without me noticing, she continued rolling the cart down the aisle.

Enter the radar of a kid who's been through

something tough.

I turned around, saw that wretched thing in MY cart, and screamed bloody murder. Now the Toys R Us employees wanted to call Child Protective Services and Animal Control.

"Get it out! Get it out! GET IT OUT!!!!!!!!"

"Okay! Okay! Okay!" my mom screamed as she threw the thing back onto the shelf like a hot potato.

Once it was out of the cart, I stopped screaming and calmed down. We were both shaken up, and we left the store with no Plan B. At this point, my mom realized that I would simply have to learn how to swim without floaty-anything. Just like they did in the colonial days. We took the "sink or swim" approach. When Kelly, Heather, or my parents were in the pool, I was right there with them, sans floaties. They held me in the water while I learned how to kick and paddle.

We spent hours in the pool together. Every day when my dad got home from work, he knew exactly where to find us. He came out to the patio and joined his little water family in the same way, every time: he walked to the deep end of the pool and reached down to splash water all over himself. Heather and Kelly swam down to the deep end and my mom brought my closer as well. Then he took a few steps back and charged into the pool, doing a full-on belly flop. We all screamed in delight as we got splashed upon impact. We were easily entertained.

I swam between my mom and dad in the shallow end while Heather and Kelly slid down the slide and perfected their flips off the diving board. When we were thoroughly water-logged, we got out of the pool and munched on whatever snack we had out on the picnic table—usually cheese puffs. Thus, those long summer days ended with us dripping wet and with fluorescent orange fingertips.

In addition to swimming, I came to love roller skating as a toddler. Turns out, I had mad roller skating skills, even at age two-and-a-half. It probably helped that I didn't have far to fall. Yes, I was a mini-roller derby queen. Kelly, Heather, and I would strap on our roller skates and skate around the garage and our driveway. Kelly could skate backwards, which always impressed the crap out of me. On special occasions, we went to a real live roller skating rink! Who knew that a disco ball and a hardwood floor could be so thrilling? The lights, the arcade games, the stale pizza—it was all so magical!

So my terrible twos were filled with swimming, roller skating, and a healthy obsession with Cabbage Patch dolls of course. I was living life as a normal kid, but my parents knew that my big surgery was just around the corner.

When I was three years old, it was finally time for my second surgery. As the date drew nearer, my parents became increasingly anxious. My mom would lose her train of thought with the slightest distraction. All she could think about was this looming monster surgery ahead of me.

About a month before the surgery, my mom and I were driving in downtown Washington DC. I was riding in the passenger seat; this was before the days of airbags and putting your kids in booster seats in the back seat until they can legally vote. Chattering away, I asked my mom a question and she turned to me and lost focus of the road ahead of her. In that split second, she ran full speed into the stopped car in front of her, which happened to contain three FBI agents. That car then rear-ended the car in front of it, which happened to contain a sheriff. Bad day. All that was missing from the scene were some nuns and an endangered animal of some sort. As it was, I'm sure my mom thought the gods were just screwing with her.

As we hit the car in front of us, the world around us felt heavier. Thankfully for me, our neighbor had lectured my mom on the need to buckle up us kids, so I was wearing a seat belt. The force of the crash propelled me into the seat belt. It all happened so fast. I looked at the glove compartment, wondering what had just happened. Then I looked to my left at my mom, and saw a horrifying scene. My mom hadn't been wearing a seatbelt, and she had been thrown forward over the steering wheel and into the windshield. She was stuck, with her head through the glass, covered in blood. I couldn't move. I couldn't turn my head. All I could do was stare at her bloody body.

One of the FBI agents rushed back to our car, saw the horrific scene, and scooped me out of the car. He stood in front of our wrecked car with me in his arms and started to direct traffic around the crash. Even though he was a perfect stranger, I clung to him for dear life. I wanted him to get us out of the street and away from the other cars. I wanted him to help my mom. All

I could do was wait and watch the chaos happening around me. I was in the eye of the tornado: safe in the arms of a stranger, but in the middle of sirens, cars, and people running everywhere.

The ambulance arrived and the EMS team immediately attended to my mom. She had miraculously survived the impact and they pulled her from the wreckage. She was awake and alert, and I watched as they loaded her on the stretcher and into the ambulance. I was passed to an EMS worker, who brought me into the ambulance with my mom. She looked at me from her stretcher and squeezed my hand, trying to reassure me that she was okay.

At the hospital we were rushed into the emergency room. The nurses and doctors checked me out and amazingly, found only bruises on my hips from the seatbelt. I stayed with my mom the whole time and stared at her from the edge of her bed. I heard the doctors saying things like "lucky to be alive." Even though I was only three, I knew that my mom should have been dead in that moment. I saw her, recover and eventually sit up. There was that feeling of relief again—I had my mom back. My dad came to the hospital to bring us home, and I was so grateful to see him because I knew that this nightmare was finally over.

We recovered from the accident just in time to face the big day of my surgery. My mom, dad, and I piled into the car and pulled into the all-too-familiar parking garage. By this time, I had been in and out of the hospital enough that I knew where we were. It got to the point where I would panic whenever we pulled into ANY parking garage, hospital or otherwise. Every time we pulled into a parking garage at a mall, I would tense up and say, "Are we at the hospital?"

"No," Mom replied, "We aren't at the hospital. We're at the mall." Whew. Close call.

This time, though, we were most assuredly at the hospital.

"Are we at the hospital?" I asked.

"Yes, honey, we are at the hospital."

"What are they going to do? Are they going to do surgery?"

Mom and Dad had prepared me for this day. I knew there was a surgery somewhere in my future and I was just dreading the day it actually happened. This was that day.

"Yes, Sweetie, this time we are here for surgery. The doctors need to fix your heart."

I got quiet. I was on alert and started watching everything around me with heightened anxiety.

We parked and got on the moving walkways. As we ascended, so did my fear. We got to the big atrium. I sat on the bucket chairs and spun. But this time it wasn't fun. All I could think about was the surgery, and no amount of spinning could take away that fear.

This time they took us to a room with a bed. This was different. We were setting up shop. The smell of the inpatient unit was different than the other clinics; it was a stronger smell, a more serious smell. We walked into the room and I saw a plastic bucket sitting on the bed, containing a pair of socks, a bar of soap, a comb, a plastic hairbrush, a tube of toothpaste, and a toothbrush. The room had blue curtains and a blue hospital blanket on the bed. While my mom helped me change into the hospital gown, the nurse checked me in. She took my blood pressure and took my temperature. The thermometer had a plastic cover on it with sharp edges that hurt my tongue.

At this point, I was pretty much ready to go to the gift shop, get my prize, and be on my way. No such luck—we had a long stay ahead of us.

After checking me in, the nurse was about to give me medications to make me less anxious. It's not uncommon for kids to get this "liquid courage" prior to surgery. For most kids, it makes them less anxious and helps them cope with scary stuff like surgery. For some reason, however, these drugs just didn't work on me; they only made me loopy enough to lose control in a bad way. They did nothing to calm my nerves—they just made me more anxious because I was still fully aware of what was happening, and I felt even more out of control than before. Because of this, my mom insisted that the nurse not give me these drugs.

Shortly after I got settled in, it was time to go back to the operating room, or the "tests" room, as everyone called it. I never liked that room, not only because it was where those nasty procedures happened, but also because I couldn't say the word "tests." I couldn't say it, so I didn't like it.

I got on the stretcher, with a white sheet and a flat pillow. I was allowed to bring one thing back with me for comfort and I chose my stuffed white cat that my neighbor had given me. As they wheeled me down the hallway—at what felt like a frenzied pace—I looked up at the ceiling to see the rectangular fluorescent lights zooming by, one at a time. I knew where I was going and I was terrified. I started to cry. Why were we going so fast? Why were the walls so white? Why did the big lights shine directly into my eyes as we wheeled past? I did not like how serious this hospital visit was.

Clutching my cat for dear life, I looked back over my shoulder to see my mom and dad, nearly running to keep up. They looked scared. They stared straight ahead and every once in a while they looked at me and said, "It's okay. You're going to be okay." I wasn't convinced. If I was going to be okay, then why did they look so worried?

When we reached the metal double doors my parents had to stay behind. They weren't allowed to come back to the operating room with me. I turned around in fear as the double doors swung closed. I couldn't see my parents anymore. I was alone back there. My tears turned into absolute hysteria as I looked around at my surroundings. The walls and ceiling weren't white anymore, they were silver. Cold. Harsh. I watched as people scurried about, some standing at a silver tray of tools, some carrying equipment around the room. They all had masks and hats on, so I couldn't even see who they were. No one seemed to notice that I was even there. They were too busy getting everything ready.

I watched and cried, still clutching my cat fearfully. Someone finally came over to talk to me. Thank God, I thought, you're here to rescue me. Now wheel me out that way, my parents are out there. They are probably wondering where I am. I should go back. Let's go.

"We need to take your pillow now," the masked man said. "You have to lie down flat."

Good luck with that one, friend. Anyone who has tried to get a hysterical toddler to lie flat knows that you have a better chance of winning the lottery and getting struck by lightning at precisely the same time. I cried even more. Now I was on a hard flat bed without even a pillow.

"It's okay," he said. "You can put your head on your cat." With that, he grabbed my cat out of my grip and smooshed it under my head. Well, that was it. First they take my pillow away and then they want me to squish my cat with my head? Poor cat! It was bad enough that I had to suffer, but the cat too? I continued crying, but I knew that I couldn't argue. This place was serious and I knew I had to follow the rules.

I lay still, feeling guilty that I was crushing my cat. Next they brought over a square, plastic box and put it over my head. This was an oxygen tent, but no one bothered to tell me that. At the top was a hole where they hooked up a hose, and I thought they were going to hose me and the cat with God knows what from above. That was the last thing I remember, so the anesthesia must have come next.

Hours later, I woke up in a completely different room. I was still encased in some sort of plastic tent, and I looked around to see a big open room. I looked to the right and saw—thank God—my parents sitting there, just staring at me. My mom was sitting in the chair, holding my hand, and my dad was sitting on the arm of the chair. As I opened my eyes, my dad tilted his head and smiled, an unspoken gesture that said, Hi there. We've been waiting for you to open those eyes. Seeing them both there was all I needed. I knew I was okay. And thank God, the cat was okay too.

I dozed off again, still groggy from the anesthesia. The next time I woke up, I had graduated from the oxygen tent. I was regaining my freedom! My mom leaned over the bed with a big smile on her face, and something cupped in her hands.

"Hi Sweetie, she said, "I have something for you."

Yes! A prize! That meant that the tough part was really over.

She brought her cupped hands closer to me and slowly opened them up. Inside was a tiny little teddy bear. He was so adorable! He was so . . .

BLECCCCHHHHHH!!!!!!

. . . covered in vomit.

And so was my mom. I cried because I felt so bad for throwing up all over my brand new teddy bear, and my mom.

"It's okay!" she said. "I'll wash him off!"

Argh. It was not my day. Just when I thought things were going my way, I puked all over the place.

In the Pediatric Intensive Care Unit (PICU), I was recovering nicely but I wasn't out of the woods yet; recovery was a long and intense road. The doctors expected me to be in the PICU for seven to ten days before moving to a step-down unit, and eventually going home. In keeping with my habit of breaking the rules, however, I was back in business after about three days. I was awake and fully aware of my surroundings, which were none too pleasant. The PICU is not a place for kids who are aware of their world. It is just plain scary. I looked around and saw machines, sedated kids, kids with tubes down their throats, kids who looked like they were dead. And all the beeping. It was non-stop. All of this was pretty much freaking me out. I needed to get out of there, but there wasn't a bed available for me on the regular units.

Mom stayed with me for the next few days and we passed the time as best we could. She held me in the rocking chair, a feat that took a team of people to accomplish because I was hooked up to more tubes than a car engine. I was like The Terminator—half machine, half human. (But not nearly as strong or Austrian).

After dinner I kept an eye on the door, knowing that any minute, my dad would walk in. Many people came in and out, nurses and doctors coming to check on me and take my vital signs. When anyone came to my hospital room door, I looked up with wide scared eyes, wondering what they were going to do. But when I saw my dad at the door, my fear instantly turned into happiness. He walked through that door at the end of his long work days and I was overjoyed. He greeted me with the biggest smile and walked over to give me monster dad hugs.

I continued to get better, and we waited for a bed to open up on a regular unit. Finally one day, the doctors came by for their daily rounding sessions. During this two-hour period, all parents had to leave the unit so they wouldn't overhear the details of the other patients. Being fully awake and aware of my surroundings, this became an upsetting time for me. Dozens of strangers came into my room and I couldn't even have my mom there with me. Enough was enough: this was not going to happen again.

"I'm not leaving her here by herself again," my mom stated very confidently to the nurse.

"No ma'am, you can't do that," the nurse said, very confidently to my mom.

"Watch me."

With that, she packed up her little Terminator, and we headed out the door.

Luckily, by this time I had rid myself of many of my tubes, so I had become more portable. Unluckily for the nurses, I had become more portable. They watched my mom as she got me ready and started for the door. They did not love my mom's stunt so much, but they also didn't try to stop her. They could have put a SWAT team in front of her, and my mom would have gotten through it. The nurse begrudgingly followed us to the playroom, where we sat and waited for my other room to become available. Going from the PICU to the playroom was like going from night to day. The PICU was intense, smelly, noisy, and the playroom was just fun. In the corner was a huge Oscar the Grouch—a grungy monster in a trash can—what more could you ask for? I toddled about from toy to toy like I was rediscovering the lost art of playing. Meanwhile, my mom and the nurse sat there together. Waiting. Amazingly, a room on the regular unit became available shortly after that; funny what a little defiance and fleeing the scene can accomplish.

I continued to recover and return to my normal self again. There were even some perks to post-surgical life, one of which was physical therapy. One of the body's ways of keeping our lungs nice and clear is by coughing and moving around, two activities that are on the 'hey, don't do that so much' list right after cardiac surgery. Without that activity, mucus can build up in the lungs and cause problems such as pneumonia. Therefore, in order to prevent post-surgical complications like pneumonia, you have to get help to break up that mucus in your lungs. How does one do that? By smacking the crap out of your back, of course! Well, more specifically, a physical therapist or respiratory therapist performs percussive therapy that involves repeatedly hitting the back with a cupped hand.

When the therapist came around to do this, all the other babies and kids cried their little eyes out, because who likes to get whacked on the back? Well, apparently I do, because every time they did it to me, I fell fast asleep. Out like a light. It was the best part of my day. Those therapists may have left a trail of tears right to my room, but when I saw them coming, it was heaven. They were like my own personal violent masseuses. It was great.

Finally I was strong enough to go home. I was discharged with strict instructions to limit my physical activity, and a schedule of follow-up appointments. During one such appointment, the nurse looked at the incision on my chest and determined that it was time to remove the surgical tape. The incision was the length of my sternum, and down the entire incision were pieces of tape, about a half-inch tall and two inches across. I wasn't too scared going into it, because it was only tape. Then she pulled the first one off and I screamed like Steve Carell from the movie, The 40-Year-Old Virgin. I don't know what sort of industrial-strength tape they used back then, but I swear it would have kept a house together. It did the trick of helping my incision close nicely, but it was shockingly painful to remove. My sudden screaming caused the nurse to stop and pull that first piece off more carefully. When it was finally removed, I breathed a sigh of relief.

And then she said, "Okay, next one."

I was so happy to have the first one off that I didn't think about the remaining 19 to come.

"No wait! Wait!" I screamed.

"We have to get it all off, Sweetie."

"No! Just wait!"

They gave me a moment to calm down.

"Okay, we need to do the next one."

Hysteria. Pulling. Pain. Why was this happening to me?

"Okay, that one's done."

Two down, 18 to go. She started in on the third one.

"No wait! Wait!" I screamed again.

Now they were on to me. I was going to delay the inevitable for as long as I could.

"Just wait!"

I tried this tactic 17 more times until we were finally

done. After the last one, I was exhausted, upset, and sore. My mom held me close to calm me down. Tape and I were not friends after that day.

After that nasty day, I resumed my normal routine of regular cardiology check-ups. Still skeptical, I continued to ask my mom every time we entered the garage, "Am I having another surgery?"

"No, Sweetie, we are just here for the kisser test and a check-up."

Thank goodness.

CHAPTER THREE

AT age three, I was on the road to recovery and things were looking up. We all took a deep breath after my open heart surgery. I had made it through the mack daddy procedure, and by all accounts thus far, it was a success. I eventually stopped asking my mom if I was having surgery every time we went to the hospital. My focus shifted from being on guard and in fear of medical procedures to actually being able to enjoy life as a kid.

In the months following surgery, I remained under physical restrictions to allow my body to heal properly, which meant no excessive activity—quite the challenge for a growing three-year-old. During those few months, I observed the world from the sidelines. I hung out with my sisters, and quietly tagged along to whatever they were doing.

Kelly, 13 at the time, was discovering the joys of being a teenager in the 1980s. She introduced me to the best pop music of the times. On many nights, I crawled onto her bed while she listened to music. Her room had bright yellow floral wallpaper that made it look like the sun threw up on the walls. She had a white, wrought iron bed with wooden globes on all the posts that popped right off. I stood on her bed and played with the wooden globes as Kelly blasted *Eye of the Tiger*. Under her tutelage, I was becoming a very cool kid.

As Kelly taught me about pop culture, Heather taught me how to focus on projects. Heather loved planning, organizing, and executing an idea. She probably could have run a business at the tender age of seven. We spent our time together building Legos. But we were not just any three- and seven-year-old kids building random block towers as high as we could. Oh no. Heather drew up architectural plans for our Lego projects, and we executed her plan with acute attention to detail. First, we brought the Lego organizer into the middle of the floor. This was a set of four drawers into which the Legos were sorted and stored. Then we placed a table mat from the dining room onto the red shag carpet. (Everyone knows that Legos can't be built on red shag carpets.) We placed the green square Lego bases on the mat, and Heather mapped out a floor plan of her dream home. She then meticulously placed each block exactly where it should go, according to her plans, and I assisted. When we were finished, we stepped back to admire our (Heather's) brilliant efforts. We were tiny, proud architects.

After two months of taking it easy, my physical restrictions were finally lifted. I had but two small requests for my celebration: my first was a roller skating party. After two long months of inactivity, I had a lot of pent-up energy. What better way to get it all out than to put me on wheels? I was like one of those toy cars that you pulled backwards and then – ZOOM! – off she goes!

I couldn't wait to brush off my skating skills. My parents planned a big party for me at the local roller rink, inviting friends and family to come celebrate with us. I awaited the day with great anticipation. Finally, I walked into the roller rink with my skates in hand. I could barely wait for my parents to pay at the window before I was off to change into my skates. Sitting on the carpeted benches, I pulled off my shoes and watched my mom as she helped me into my skates. I hobbled over to the entrance of the rink and waited for my chance. Getting onto a roller skating rink is like merging onto a busy highway. I waited for the swarms of people to offer an opening, and then stepped onto the rink. I clung to the wall for a few steps, to build up my confidence, and then made my way into the center of the ring. There, I circled the track again and again to the tunes of many an 80s hair band ballad. I was finally free to be a normal kid again!

Kelly and Heather were also expert skaters. I latched onto them on some laps so they could pull me around the track even faster. The whole day was full of fun and celebration. It marked a monumental step in my recovery. We all knew that the tough stuff was behind us now, and the rest of my life would be smooth sailing.

My second request was a pair of Jordache jeans.

Anyone who remembers the 1980s knows the wonderment of Jordache jeans. They were the ultimate in denim wear and their logo was a horse – any girl's dream. I had to have them. Unfortunately, Jordache didn't make a toddler collection, but that didn't stop me; I still had to have my Jordaches. It didn't matter that I was swimming in my oversized new duds, or that my mom had to roll the cuffs up nine inches. I had my Jordache jeans and a matching sweatshirt with the Jordache horse, so I was in heaven. I felt so proud and grown up. I wore those jeans everywhere, and made my mom take lots of pictures of me wearing them. My pose had to be perfect, because you had to see the horse logo on the butt, and I also had to look at the camera. This resulted in a series of shots with me looking over my shoulder with my hand on my hiney, highlighting the logo. I taught Tyra Banks everything she knows.

Even at the age of three, I knew that a girl had to look her best, which, incidentally, was a big reason why I didn't join the Brownies years later. Heather and Kelly were both active members of the Brownies and my mom was their troop leader. I tagged along on day trips, to meetings, parties, cookie sales, and all sorts of organized fun. When Heather graduated from the Brownies, I still had one more year before I was old enough to be a Brownie, so my mom stayed on as troop leader. I continued to participate as a non-official member, loving every minute of it, and the day finally came when I was old enough to make it official.

"Jamie, guess what," my mom said.

"What?"

"You're old enough to join the Brownies for real! We can sign you up and you can be a real Brownie."

"No way."

"What?"

"I don't want to be a Brownie."

My mom was fairly perplexed by this. Why didn't I want to be a Brownie when I'd loved tagging along with her all this time?

"Why not?"

"Because I don't want to sit in that dumb circle and I'm not wearing that ugly brown outfit."

My mom promptly quit as Brownie leader, and wondered why I had wasted the last year of her life. It's kind of her fault, though; she raised an independent kid with good fashion sense. What did she expect?

After my heart surgery, nothing stopped me. I had all the energy of a normal kid and loved what most little girls did: hanging out with my big sisters, getting new Cabbage Patch Kids, building Legos, and playing with people's hair. As a kid, I was obsessed with long hair. I had a cropped 'do that almost made me look like a mini-Beatles impersonator. I wanted long hair so badly, though, that I went about my day with a striped dishtowel on my head. Fake it 'til you make it, I guess. It did the trick as a substitute until my real hair grew. During this time, my idol was Crystal Gayle, the country singer with long, flowing locks down to her ankles. My mom listened to her album while she worked around the house, and I just stared at the cover as I listened to "Don't it Make My Brown Eyes Blue." I coveted her hair almost like a crazed little stalker.

My obsession didn't stop there, either. One day my mom took me shopping at a department store. She was looking through racks of clothes and I was just tagging along, trying to entertain myself. A few minutes passed and my mom realized that it was suddenly very quiet. Sure enough, she looked down, and I was nowhere to be found. She called my name and searched the nearby area. A few panic-stricken moments later, she found me. I was perfectly content, brushing the hair of a mannequin positioned low to the ground, and therefore fully accessible to me. My mom scolded me for messing with the store display, but I really didn't think I had done anything wrong. If anything, I was doing the store personnel a favor by helping them maintain their lovely displays. Looking back, it was a little creepy of me to be that obsessed with long hair. Thank God we didn't have the Internet back then—I would have had my own chat room at age five.

Apart from the slightly odd hair obsession, I continued through my young school age years like most kids do. The repair on my heart was holding up very well, and my medical life consisted of the occasional check-up. My only physical limitation was that I didn't have endless stamina. Luckily, I wasn't training for any marathons so it worked out okay. Life was good, and I was in the clear.

When I turned four, it was time to enter pre-school. Until then, my experience with school was of dropping off and picking up Heather from Montessori school. By all accounts, it was a pretty cool place with plenty of things to do. The people seemed nice enough. I could probably handle something like this.

For the first time, I joined in on the "first day of school" picture on our front porch, and we loaded into the car. Heather was off to her classroom and my mom and I started walking to my classroom. I walked in to see a whole mess of kids and several teachers milling about. It was pretty intimidating, so I stuck close to my mom. One of the teachers walked up to us to welcome me to the class.

"Hi Jamie!"

Back off, lady. I'm just checking things out.

"Sweetie, why don't you go play with the other kids and I'll be back later to pick you up," my mom said, as if it was no big deal.

Forget that. No way.

I didn't say anything, but clung to my mom's leg. They were going to have to pry me off if they wanted me to stay there. I was expecting my mom to take one look at how upset I was, pick me up, and head out the door, saying, "Thank you anyway," to the teacher.

Not so much. Apparently, my mom was also all for the idea of my staying there without her. ALL DAY. BY MYSELF.

Once I realized that I wasn't going home with my mom, I did what every other logical four-year-old would have done: I had a meltdown. God, you would have thought they were trying to put floaties on my arms.

My mom looked at me with sad eyes and said, "You'll be just fine. You'll have fun! And when you are done, you will get to go see Kelly at her locker, and then I'll pick you up." The fact that Kelly's middle school was also in the same building gave me no comfort. She couldn't help me. I was on my own. Left to fend for myself.

My mom finally left and I sobbed as she walked out the door. So this was my life now. No more coddling. I had to take care of myself now.

My crying went from hysterical to just weepy, and I still wanted nothing to do with pre-school. The teacher brought me over to story time and showed me the carpet squares. "You can pick any one you want," she said.

I pick the one in my mom's car.

I begrudgingly picked a red one and sat down with the other kids. By the end of the day, I ended up playing with some of the toys and had a small amount of fun. When it was all over, the teacher took me to Kelly's locker to find her. I was so happy to see her! When Mom came to get me, I breathed a sigh of relief and hopped into the car. Thank God that was over.

The next day, we piled into the car again. We were going back to that place?! Are you kidding me? One day was traumatic enough. Hadn't we all learned our lesson from that wretched experience? Apparently not, because here we went again.

This time, my tears started the moment we entered the room. The teacher looked at my mom like, Oh hi. You're back. Great.

"Hi Jamie," she said.

Beat it! I thought.

My mom and the teacher made the transition faster

this time; she gave me a big hug and quickly left the room.

I cried. And cried. I picked up my stupid red carpet square and sat down in misery with the other kids, who, by the way, didn't seem to realize what an awful place this was. They were perfectly happy. Didn't they know that their parents weren't there? Dumb kids.

When my mom picked me up that day, the teacher told her that it had taken me a long time to calm down again. "Maybe you should think about starting off with only three days a week," she said. Because I need at least two days during the week when I don't hate my job, she thought.

"Okay, that's a good idea. We'll try that."

From there, we eased into preschool a little more gradually. I finally got to the point where I didn't cry, and eventually even enjoyed myself the whole day. It may have had something to do with the fact that one of the teachers gave me chocolate gum; when in doubt, bribery works.

The next couple of years of school were much less traumatic. Starting in kindergarten, I got to choose a backpack, a lunch box, and school supplies. That made everything better. I got to see Heather in the hallways of school when I was in second grade. Knowing one of the upperclassmen (a fourth grader) always made me feel cool. By this time, Kelly was in high school, and I still got to go see her at her locker. This was such fun, with the exception of her one friend who smothered me with overzealous affection. She must not have had a little sister of her own, because every time she saw me, so attacked me like that aunt who squeezes your cheeks way too hard. I loved attention, but man, she needed to ease up. I was pretty tiny for my age, and I think she thought I was her own little Polly Pocket. Not fun. I saw her coming and tried to escape before she picked me up. I never fully evaded her, though, and had to withstand the smothering.

My life was punctuated with cardiology check-ups, but for the most part I was living a normal life. During the winter, Kelly, Heather, and I spent hours in the snow, building snowmen and forts. Heather was the architect of the forts, of course. When the weather warmed up, we swapped our snowsuits and moonboots for bikes and bathing suits. My dad bought a four-wheeler and we drove around in the field behind our house. I strapped on the big clunky helmet and helped steer.

My dad built us a clubhouse above our storage shed— the best clubhouse ever. It had a balcony that looked out over our yard. It was also carpeted and had a stained glass window. We played in style. My dad was a glazier and stained glass artist, and owned a glass company. Therefore, our house and our clubhouse were adorned with amazing works of stained glass art.

I loved watching my dad work on his projects. When we visited him at work, I looked through all his colored glass and he showed me what he was working on. Under strict instructions to not touch anything, I watched him cut huge pieces of glass and break them apart like plastic. He was a pro. He let me practice on scrap pieces of glass next to him. Every once in a while, he cut himself and took out his first aid kit. And by first aid kit, I mean shoe box with paper towels and duct tape. A little deep tissue gash never hurt anyone. So what if it severed the nerves? Just put an extra layer of paper towels on it.

He taught us all how to cut glass, and we continued our apprenticeship at home in his workshop. Kelly helped him with his more complicated projects by wrapping the small pieces of glass with lead strips to be soldered together. I played with the soldering gun and melted metal into puddles. When we needed a break from that, we went outside to play on his glass truck. It was a pickup truck with tall racks on each side of the bed – perfect for climbing. It was like a jungle gym on wheels over a bed of broken glass.

Those days filled with power tools and shards of glass were the best. We were the only three kids in the neighborhood who could cut glass, which could have proven to be a very useful skill given the direction our neighborhood was going. Our very nice suburban neighborhood was turning a little shady. No longer could we stay out until dark, puttering around outside, riding bikes around the whole neighborhood. A family moved in down the block and started causing a little trouble. Heather was out playing one day and when she came back home, she was being followed by a group of kids who meant trouble. Kelly and I were out on the lawn and we saw the group approaching. They were messing with Heather, and pushed her down on the driveway. Kelly ran over to yell at them and make them leave. After that incident, we knew to beware of this group of kids. For the first time ever, we had to watch our backs, and my parents knew we had a problem. Before we had to use our glass cutting skills to make homemade shanks for protection, my parents decided that it was time to move.

We often went on camping trips—yuck—to Pennsylvania. This was what my parents referred to as a "vacation." They used that term loosely. We had a pop-up camper that we towed to the campsite. There, we had to assemble our shelter. It was a nightmare. My parents so desperately wanted us to love it, but I wanted nothing to do with it. If you have to walk a mile in the cold through the woods to go to the bathroom in the middle of the night, then that is not a vacation. Even prisoners have bathrooms right there in their cells. If this was supposed to build character, then it did the trick; my character was shaping up to be one that hated camping.

Still, my parents loved it. It was "quality time." "As a family." Yeah, well you know what else offers quality time? Hotels.

Enamored with the setting and the relaxed pace of being in the country, my parents started looked for a place for us there. They found a 6-acre plot of land just a mile from their beloved campground, nestled in the woods by a creek. They started to build our dream home there, and we actually had loads of fun exploring the woods and playing in the creek. It was also nice not to worry about getting attacked by neighborhood hoodlums. There, all we had to worry about was the mosquitoes. And the best part? Our new house would have plumbing. No more camping! Hallelujah.

Of course, moving to Pennsylvania also meant leaving our home in Maryland. We were leaving our pool, our clubhouse, and our best friends who lived down the street. No longer would we get to see them every day. On the last move-out day, we piled the last of our belongings, including our dog Floppy and our cat Charlie, into our red Volvo station wagon. I sat next to Charlie in his cat carrier and watched out the back window as our house got smaller and smaller. We were moving on to the next phase of our lives, having no idea what waited for us on the road ahead.

My dad had opened his glass company in Maryland years before, and he still owned and operated it after we moved. Every day he drove two hours each way, waking up at three in the morning, driving down to his shop, and taking a nap on his workbench until he opened the shop. At the end of the day, he closed up at five and made the long trip home to us. He did this every day, but sometimes broke up the week by staying one night at the Econo Lodge by his shop. When he did this, he always came home with a bag of Raisinets from the bulk section of the grocery store. He never took a sick day. Day after day, week after week, he did this. He was always in a good mood and happy to see us when he got home, even though he was exhausted. We greeted him at the door with big hugs, having missed him all day. He didn't put in these long hours because he loved the job; he did it for us, so we could have the security of his business and our new life in Gettysburg.

I was busy acclimating to third grade in a brand new

school with brand new classmates. I had a mullet. It was 1987, people, give a girl a break. Heather was starting middle school, and Kelly was going into her first year of college. I made fast friends with my classmates, and even had a little boyfriend in my class. We played together at recess, and he put my chair up on my desk for me every day after school. Hence, he was my boyfriend.

The new house offered a whole new set of adventures. Heather and I explored the woods and climbed all over the rocks by the creek. We also became expert crayfish catchers. We put on our rubber boots and traipsed down to the creek with nets and buckets. After filling up our buckets with a fresh haul, we dumped the pile of crayfish back into the creek. Poor crayfish. They probably liked it much better before we moved in.

I often snuggled with my dad on his leather chair, watching TV. Finding a western movie on TV was like hitting the jackpot for my dad. Every once in a while, though, I convinced him to watch something else and that something else was usually Star Wars. One afternoon, we were watching The Empire Strikes Back. Even though we could recite the lines of all three original movies, we still watched with rapt attention.

Luke Skywalker had just escaped the Snow Creature's deadly capture, and was staggering around the icy tundra on Planet Hoth. He was weak and confused. Thanks to the power of the Force (or some kind of intergalactic hallucinogen), Luke saw his fallen mentor Obi Wan (Ben) Kenobi. After a brief chat with his apparition friend, Luke collapsed, powerless against the frigid temperatures. Just then, like a knight in shining armor, Han Solo came over the ridge on his Tauntaun to rescue Luke. The Tauntaun was no match for the cold, and he fell over dead. Next came my favorite part. Han sliced open the belly of the Tauntaun, spilling its guts out all over the snow. Then he smushed Luke inside the gutted beast to keep him warm for the night.

Disgusting.

At this point, my dad jumped in to offer some good fatherly advice. "You know, if that Tauntaun was dead, he wouldn't be able to generate body heat. So he wouldn't keep Luke warm at all. He would still die of exposure."

"Oh," I said.

"So if you are ever stranded outside with a dead animal, it won't help you to cut it open and crawl inside."

"Okay," I said, dutifully.

My dad always wanted us to be prepared. And now I know that if I am ever stranded on the icy planet of Hoth, I won't even bother slicing open my dead Tauntaun. It won't save me.

CHAPTER FOUR

THREE years after my surgery, my mom got a phone call from my doctor. "Hello ma'am. How's Jamie doing?" he asked.

"She's fine, thank you," Mom replied.

"That's good to hear. Well, I'm calling because there is something we need to talk about."

He continued on to tell my mom that there had been advances in medicine that led to the discovery of new diseases. "You may have heard of the disease called AIDS."

"Yes."

"We are now aware of the presence of AIDS, and there have been tests developed to screen blood products for the virus that causes AIDS, called HIV. Five years ago, when Jamie had her surgery, that test didn't exist. As you know, Jamie received a blood transfusion during her surgery."

"Yes . . ."

"Since that blood wasn't screened, there is a very slight possibility that it was infected with the HIV virus. It's very unlikely, but we are informing everyone who had a blood transfusion during that time about this possibility."

"What should we do?" my mom asked.

"Well, has Jamie been healthy since her heart surgery?"

"Yes. She's made a great recovery. Her cardiac symptoms subsided, and she's been an active little girl. She's been very healthy."

"Has she ever gotten sick in the last five years?" he asked.

"Rarely. She'll get a cold now and then, but nothing out of the ordinary. She didn't even get chickenpox when her sister got it. I even had her play with her sister while she was sick so she would get it early and have it out of the way, but she never got it."

"Then she's probably fine. You probably have nothing to worry about," he said.

"Should we get her tested?" Mom asked.

"It's up to you. It's very unlikely that she has it, and she probably would have been very sick if she did have it. You're probably fine to not even worry about getting her tested."

My mom hung up and talked to my dad about the doctor's news. They discussed whether or not they should get me tested, and decided that I was probably fine. I had gotten poked and prodded so much growing up, and they didn't want to make me get poked again if I really didn't have to.

Shortly after that phone call, I came home from school with a scratchy throat. It was a pretty common affliction for a school kid, but my mom took me to the doctor after it didn't go away on its own. The doctor diagnosed me with strep throat. He sent us home with a prescription for antibiotics, and it went away. A few weeks later, I came home again with a sore throat. We went back to the doctor, who diagnosed me again with strep throat, and sent me home once again with antibiotics. A few weeks later, I came home with another scratchy throat. This was getting annoying. Sure enough, I had round three of strep throat.

For me, this was just a pain to be getting sick again and again. For my parents, though, this was an alarming sign that they needed to investigate. My mom called my doctor in Maryland to tell them about my recurrence of strep throat. He said it could be a fluke, but just to be safe, I should probably get tested.

My mom made the appointment.

"Hey Sweetie," she told me, "we have to go down to the hospital to get a blood test."

Boo. To me, it was just another blood test. I never liked them, but I was fairly used to them at this point. I didn't think anything about it; we had gone to the hospital so many times before for check-ups that I just thought this was another one of those.

A couple of weeks after my blood test, my mom got a phone call from the doctor. She answered the phone and the doctor did his best to delay the inevitable; he went around in circles, saying anything but what he actually called to say. Finally, he said it.

"The test is positive. You should come down here so we can talk about what this means."

She hung up the phone, having just learned that her daughter had a deadly disease, and she had no one to tell. My dad was at work, and she didn't dare tell any of our new acquaintances, or even her old friends.

My mom drove to the doctor's office to talk about this news. She walked in to find him sitting at his desk. He greeted her and proceeded to recline in his chair with his hands interlocked behind his head, as if he were about to start talking to my mom about summer vacations.

"Jamie's test came back positive," he began. "She has, at best, two years to live. If I were you, I would enjoy your time with her while you can."

That was it. No sitting down next to my mom. No offering her tissues. It was the ultimate violation of the Rules of Human Decency. It was only because my mom was in a state of utter shock that he made it out of that meeting alive. Ever heard of a mama bear? Think of that times a million—that is what he would have dealt with had she had all of her wits about her.

She got up, stunned, and walked out of the office. When she got home, she told my dad what the doctor said; neither of them knew what it meant for us, but they knew it was serious.

"What should we tell her?" my mom asked.

"We can't tell her anything," my dad replied. "She won't understand and it will only scare her."

"We have to tell her something."

"No, we can't scare her."

"She's a smart kid. She's going to know something's wrong when she starts getting sick more and more often, and doesn't get any better. We're going to have to be there for her when she dies, and we can't not tell her anything!"

My dad wanted to protect me from the truth, but mom convinced him that they would have to tell me something. Then they had my sisters to think about. How on earth were they going to tell Heather and Kelly that their little sister was going to get sick very quickly and probably die?

Kelly was in the middle of final exams, so they decided that it was not the best time to tell her. My mom talked to the staff at the hospital and made arrangements to bring Heather and me in for the conversation.

We piled into the car. "Girls, we are going to the hospital."

"How come?" I asked. At this point, I knew that I had a problem with my heart that required me to go in for frequent check-ups. I figured it was another one of those check-ups.

"We aren't going to do any tests today. We are just going to have a talk," she said.

Panic set in. This could only mean that my worst fear was coming true. They were going to tell me I had to have another heart surgery, and the thought terrified me. I was a little ball of nerves from that point forward.

"Do I have to have another heart surgery?" I asked her. Let's just cut to the chase, lady. Tell me like it is.

"No, you don't have to have another surgery. We'll

talk about everything when we get there."

Mmmmm hmmmmm. I was still suspicious.

We parked in the dreaded parking garage and took the long slanted moving walkway into the all-too-familiar hospital atrium. Dottie, one of my favorite nurses, met us there and took us into a small room with white walls. Heather waited outside in the waiting room.

We sat down and Dottie started talking.

"Jamie, there is something we need to tell you."

"Do I have to have another heart surgery?"

"No. We did a blood test that showed that you have a bug in your blood."

"Does it have to do with my heart?" I asked.

"No."

"Is there something else wrong with my heart?"

"No."

"Do I have to get another heart surgery?" I had to be absolutely sure of this one.

"No."

That was all I needed to hear. As long as I didn't need another surgery, I was happy as a clam.

"Is that it?" I asked.

"Yes. Do you have any questions?"

"No," I replied. I already had the answer I needed— no heart surgery. I was quite relieved, and quite ready to go. I was done. I didn't want to hear anything else. I felt a great rush of relief, thinking that I had just dodged a bullet by avoiding heart surgery. A bug in my blood? I could handle that. I walked out of that room perfectly content with life and not needing to know anything else that day.

Their job wasn't done, however. Heather was out in the waiting room, and it was her turn to go in for a talk. They took me out of the room and I went with another one of my favorite nurses to hang out while they talked to Heather.

It's all good, I mentally told Heather. You'll do fine. And good news: I don't have to have heart surgery.

Heather, being 12 years old, was at an age where she could process more information. My mom knew they would have to be very upfront with her. Heather was also our resident worrier in the family, and they knew that she would not be able to pass it off like I did. Heather was the queen of "what if"—a true information seeker.

"Heather, we have something to tell you about Jamie. When she had her heart surgery, she got a blood transfusion. We didn't know it at the time, but that blood was infected with HIV, the virus that causes AIDS. Jamie has this virus now, and it's very serious. There aren't any medicines we can give her. She's probably going to get very sick in the next couple of years, and she's not going to survive it."

Heather sobbed and sobbed. While I was outside, blissfully unaware of the reality of what they had just told us, Heather got it.

After she had gotten her tears out, my mom said to her, "Now Heather, here is the hardest thing. Jamie doesn't really know what this means for her, and we can't tell her until she's ready to hear it. She's not ready yet, so we can't cry in front of her."

Heather nodded. She understood.

Meanwhile, in oblivious-land, I was happily playing with the nurse. Their talk was taking a lot longer than mine, I noticed. When they finally came out of the room, I happily rejoined them. They seemed quiet.

Heather walked up to me, put her arm around my shoulder and said, "Hey kid, you wanna go to the gift shop?" without blinking an eye.

Yes! Finally, we got to the fun part of the day!

After that day at the hospital, life went on just the same for me. In my mind, nothing had changed. I had a bug in my blood, so what? I felt fine, and I didn't have to have surgery to fix it, so things were good.

When Kelly was done with her finals, my mom had the same conversation with her, explaining that she couldn't say anything to me about it.

My family now faced a new life with a daughter, a sister, who would die soon. There was nothing anyone could do for me. There were no medications for kids with HIV in 1987. The only sure thing that people knew about HIV was that if you had it, you were going to die. My parents and my sisters watched me closely, wondering when I would start to get sick, and when I would start asking questions. Knowing that at some point I would get sick, my mom put me on a waiting list for any upcoming pediatric HIV protocols at the National Institutes of Health (NIH). It was the only hint of treatment that was available at the time.

Soon after that day at the hospital, we took a family vacation to the Grand Canyon. We stayed in a little resort in the woods. (More vacations in the woods? Really?) Every morning we walked outside and fed the deer, who were so used to tourists that they came right up to us. Seeing the Grand Canyon for the first time was incredible. I had never seen anything that huge before in my life. It wasn't so incredible for Heather, who in addition to being our worrier, was afraid of heights. Poor kid. If I wandered too close to the edge—within 100 yards—she freaked out and yelled at me to come back. She probably would have been quite content with a nice coffee table book about the Grand Canyon, versus actually being there.

While we were there, we took a rafting trip down the Colorado River. There, we could enjoy the canyon from below, which made Heather much happier. We loaded onto a pontoon boat, clad in dirty yellow life vests, and started down the river. We floated in the vast expanse of the river, banked against the towering orange and red walls of the canyon. I sat with Kelly and Heather on the edge of the boat, dipping my feet into the freezing cold water to cool off from the sweltering heat. We stopped for lunch at a flat part of the bank and hopped out of the boat into the water, which was like jumping into a vat of ice water. My mom wanted to get a picture of each of us in the water, but it was too cold to stay in for more than a few moments. So we ran into the water, smiled for the picture, and ran out before our toes got numb.

Soon after we got back from the Grand Canyon, we planned a trip to England, where my dad grew up. To prepare for the trip, my mom took us out shopping for our travel clothes. Yes, we were like the Von Trapp family, but flying was a formal affair back then. Now, it's a slumber party. (I'm sorry. I know you're planning to nap on the plane, but Sponge Bob pajama pants? Really? How about some yoga pants or something?) The other amazing thing about our flights: hot meals. Free ones. It was the most disgusting Salisbury steak ever created, but it came on its own little tray, so I thought it was the coolest thing ever.

My parents packed bags of activities to keep us busy on the long flights. This kept us occupied, and prevented us from bugging the other passengers. When we boarded one flight to England, a man sat down next to Heather and me. We liked to sit with each other because we could play together and it made us feel cool and responsible. Our parents were sitting two feet away, but still. I'm sure this man was thrilled to be sitting next to two kids. Turns out though, we were always well-behaved, and kept to ourselves. Heather and I played our travel games—magnetic checkers, travel Yahtzee. This guy read his book and glanced at us from time to time.

Once he ascertained that we weren't hyperactive or whiny or slobbery, he actually started talking to us. "That's a cool game."

"Thanks," Heather said.

"Thanks," I said, leaning over Heather to talk to him. "You can play if you want."

"Okay."

He joined in our game of Yahtzee.

"Are you guys going on vacation?"

"Yeah," I said. "Our dad is from England, so we're going on vacation there."

"That's pretty cool."

"Yeah."

We continued playing Yahtzee. Our parents glanced over at us to make sure the guy didn't look like a pedophile. So far, so good.

We chatted with our airplane buddy as we wrapped up the game and got ready for our meal tray. The schlopp they put before us looked so delicious. Maybe it was the altitude, but it felt like gourmet dining.

I started to eat my salad, and pushed around my cherry tomato. I was not a fan. I looked over at Airplane Guy and he was devouring his salad, tomato and all.

"Hey. Do you want my tomato?" I asked.

The guy looked at me, perplexed, like he was trying to figure me out. He stared at me for a few seconds, contemplating.

"Sure," he said.

I reached across Heather with my bowl and he scooped it off.

"Thanks," he said.

"Sure."

We ate in silence for a few moments.

Then he leaned over to me.

"You want my cookie?" he asked me.

"Sure. Thanks."

"No problem."

Heather, the utter introvert that she was, was quite ready for our little bartering session to be over. I was just happy that I had a new friend who gave me cookies. When we landed in England, I said farewell to Airplane Guy, and we started our adventures.

We arrived at our rented cottage in Cirencester, England, and Heather and I ran up the four flights of stairs to claim our bedrooms and explore the house. When we were settled in, we all walked outside to explore the little town. Across the street were a church and a duck pond. There was a bakery a few doors down that also sold fresh milk in bottles. To my dad's delight, we found a fish 'n chips shop just around the corner. It was so quaint, like England's Little House on the Prairie.

Every morning, we started off early and took long drives to see cathedrals, castles, and other historical landmarks. Heather and I brought books to read in the car, but we got in trouble for reading them. Yes. We were told not to read. "Stop reading your books, girls!" they hollered. "Look at the scenery!" Forced tourism at its best.

On our low-key days, we stayed in town and did my favorite activity: feeding the ducks and geese. We bought day-old bread from the bakery for a cheap price, and then we walked across the street to the duck pond. Those birds were smart. They knew that people came there to feed them, and they came right up to us to get their bounty. They were all pretty fat.

As they swarmed us like rabid raccoons, I saw one funny-looking goose hanging out at the back. He always got pushed aside by the other bullies, and never got any bread. He had a wonky foot that made him wobble when he walked, and his feathers were a mess. I'd throw some bread to him and another bird would trample him to steal it. It was pathetic.

While Heather distracted the flock, I walked over to this goose to give him his own stash of bread. He gobbled it up. That goose was my best friend for the rest of our trip. I named him Wobbles. Every time we came to the pond, Wobbles walked right up to me to get his treats. He just needed a little special attention.

The other important lesson I learned on this trip was that swans, although beautiful, are mean sons of bitches. They look so graceful and elegant until they came charging towards you with the fury of a mountain lion. They soon learned that I fed Wobbles away from the crowd, and thought, *Perfect, a disabled goose and a pipsqueak kid.* This will be a piece of cake. Yeah, they came at me good. I learned that the best strategy to avoid getting my eyes pecked out by the beastly swans was to run like a coward. My dad often had to intervene and shoo away the swans before they got me. So it was a really educational trip; I learned all about British history, as well as valuable self-defense skills when faced with a greedy swan.

Our next trip was a cruise through the Hawaiian Islands. I was beginning to love these family adventures! We had never been on a cruise before, and never been to Hawaii, so we all looked forward to this trip with great anticipation. The cruise ship had a clubhouse for the kids (to give parents a break), which had its own bar-style soda dispenser. I drank so much soda, just because I could. They also had kid activities in the pool, like Spoon Toss. This was a very complicated game in which the lifeguard threw a bucket of spoons in the pool and we dove in to retrieve them all. We were easily entertained.

Self-serve sodas and diving for dirty silverware were only the beginning of our adventures, though. We docked and explored what the islands had to offer. We hopped on a tour bus and drove up to the site of a recent lava flow. When we got off the bus, it was like we were on another planet; the ground beneath us was black, hardened lava, still in the smooth shape of its flow. Small pockets of it were still steaming. A few yards away, behind yellow caution tape, the lava still glowed red and emitted heat waves.

Next, we rented a car and drove to the famous black sand beach. The sand was actually lava that had been crumbled into sand when it reached the shore. It was amazing. Tourists often took some of the sand and bigger chunks of lava home as souvenirs. The locals warned us against doing this, because they said it brought bad luck to whomever took it home. We thought that was just a hokey legend that the locals told dumb tourists to keep them from stealing all their sand and rocks, so we each picked up a small rock and a handful of sand and put it in a plastic bag to take home.

When we boarded the ship, the staff asked us how our day was.

"It was great!" my mom said. "We took a tour to the lava flow and we saw the black sand beach."

"Did you pick up any lava rocks?"

Are you kidding? All these people must have been

scripted to say this to protect their precious lava rocks.

"We did." My mom couldn't flat-out lie.

"Have you heard that's bad luck? I wouldn't take it off the island if I were you. The post office in this town has piles of packages filled with lava rocks that people have sent back because they have been cursed by taking them home."

For real?

"That's good to know. Thanks," my mom said.

We then promptly walked to the side of the ship, threw our rocks back into the water, and dumped our bags of sand overboard. We did not need to tempt fate. Hokey legend or not, we were in no position to take chances.

The next stop on our trip was to see Pearl Harbor on the island of Oahu. The pristine white memorial built over the sunken ship was breathtaking. I stared over the side of the memorial to see the U.S.S. Arizona sitting right beneath us. We wandered through the museum and saw the many artifacts that were pulled up, including the anchor that was as big as a truck. My dad, a military history buff, read every single plaque on the exhibits. We spent a lot of time there.

Back on board, we soaked up the sun and enjoyed the perks of cruise life. After spoon diving and soda pouring, we partook in the grand American tradition— the midnight buffet. You haven't lived until you have gorged on a midnight buffet. It was so elaborately laid out that they had a preliminary viewing, where everyone walked through the buffet and looked at it before taking any food. I'd never seen a swan carved out of lard before, and I was very thankful that this swan wasn't going to peck my eyes out. There were intricate ice sculptures and fruit carved into scenic dioramas. After we feasted on the luxurious spread, we went to bed and let the food coma set in.

We came home from that trip exhilarated and already making plans to go back. That buffet was well worth the 10 hours of travel time.

I was loving life and filling my room with all kinds of tacky souvenirs. Why had we never gone on vacations like this before? This was awesome! We continued on this vacation rampage and went on a couple of trips per year, usually alternating between Hawaii and England.

Meanwhile, I was still oblivious my disease. My parents watched me closely when HIV or AIDS was mentioned on TV, and I didn't even blink. I never once asked about the "bug in my blood." I continued on with my cardiac check-ups, and life went on as usual. I got sick from time to time, but I never thought anything about it. I just liked the days off of school.

Two years later, when I was 10 years old, a new protocol opened up at NIH for a Phase I clinical drug trial for pediatric HIV. Since I had been on the waiting list, the researcher called my mom to tell her I could join the protocol, if I met the criteria.

"What would this involve?" my mom asked.

"We would bring Jamie in for some lab work and go over her history to see if she fits the criteria for the protocol. Assuming she does, we'll go over all of the details of what you would need to do. Basically, we would start off by doing two days of testing to get some baseline data on her."

"What kind of tests would you have to do?"

"We would do an MRI, CT scan, lumbar puncture, echocardiogram, EKG, chest x-ray and lab work. We would do some additional testing with the occupational therapy, physical therapy, optometry, and neuropsychology departments."

"This is the only protocol available, right?" she asked.

"Yes, that's right."

"Well, this sounds like the best and only option for her. What do we do next?"

My mom talked to my dad about this protocol and what it would mean for me. "We have an appointment to get the initial testing done. But we have to tell her what we are doing," she said.

"What do you mean? She knows that she has something besides her heart problem. Why would we want to scare her?"

"Well, she'll be going to a new hospital, going through tons of testing, and she's going to see posters about AIDS all over the clinic. She's going to start asking questions and I think we should tell her now before she gets confused."

They agreed that they had to tell me in no uncertain terms that I was HIV positive. They knew they couldn't smoke this one by me without telling me what was really going on.

My mom and I headed back to the hospital to have another talk. We pulled into the parking garage and I asked my standard set of questions.

"What are we here for?"

"We're just going to talk."

"Do I have to have another heart surgery?"

"No."

Phew.

We hopped on to the moving walkway, entered the atrium, and found my friend Dottie, who took us to a different room this time. This one was much cozier, and we all sat down on couches.

This again? I was thinking. Didn't we already do this? I have a bug in my blood; I get it. Why are we sitting here again?

"Jamie, do you remember when we talked about you having a bug in your blood?" Dottie said.

"Yes."

"That bug is called HIV."

"Okay," I said. *I have no idea what that means*, I thought.

Dottie continued, "HIV is the virus that causes AIDS."

That was a word I knew. There was no sugar coating this anymore; I got it when she said AIDS. From then on, I only remember vague hints of the rest of the conversation.

I was scared.

I cried.

Was I going to die? People with AIDS died.

"You have had this since your surgery, and have stayed pretty healthy growing up. We want you to stay healthy, though, and there is another hospital where we can help you do that."

"I have to go to a new hospital?"

"Yes," my mom piped in. "I've talked to them and they are very nice."

"This place also has medicines you can take that will hopefully keep you healthy," Dottie continued.

I did not want to go to a new hospital that I knew nothing about, but I knew I didn't have a choice.

I cried from fear of getting sick. I cried about having to go to a new hospital. There was a lot to cry about that day. When I calmed down, my mom said, "I know this is hard to hear, Sweetie, but we are going to see what this hospital can do for you, okay?"

"Okay," I said.

They both hugged me hard.

"Okay, mom?" I said. "You can tell Heather and Kelly now."

"They already know."

For real? I'm always the last to know things. How come I didn't know when they already did? How come I never saw them cry about it? What had Heather and Kelly thought all this time? Did they think that I was going to die?

"Were they upset?"

"Yes, they were very upset, but they know that you have always been strong and that we are going to do everything we can to keep you healthy."

"Okay."

I walked out of that room not feeling hopeless or depressed. I didn't think my life was over. I knew it was serious, but I held out hope that these medicines would work. The only way to go forward was to do so optimistically.

Dottie, my mom, and I walked down the big orange hallway, linked arms and started skipping, like Dorothy and her friends in The Wizard of Oz. We were off to see the Wizard all right, and none of us knew what that meant. But that didn't stop us from skipping along the way. If you had seen us skipping down the hall, arm in arm that day, you wouldn't have guessed at the conversation that had just taken place.

This was symbolic of my entire experience of living with HIV, to that point. I was surrounded by people who told me the truth and answered my questions honestly—even the tough ones—and still carried me forward with hope.

In the days that followed, I processed through this new life of mine and relied on my parents for the answers. Being the kind of kid who needed to know what was going on, I didn't hold back. One afternoon, my mom and I were sitting on Mom and Dad's bed, nestled in the mauve, floral-patterned (eek!) bedspread and pillows.

"What kind of medicine am I going to have to take?" I asked.

"It's called DDI."

"Do I have to get shots?"

"The medicine is in liquid form, so you just have to drink it. There will be times, though, that they will have to take your blood when we visit the hospital."

"How come?"

"This is how they are going to see how well the

medicine is working."

"Am I going to die?"

She looked at me and said, "I don't know honey."

She didn't say, 'No, honey, that's not going to happen,' or 'No, you're going to be just fine.' She was honest with me. At that moment, it became very real to me that we didn't know what my future held, but that we would get through it together. I wasn't devastated. I wasn't hysterical. I was becoming at peace with it.

"If I die, I want Heather to have the CD player in my room."

She hugged me close. "Sweetie, hopefully these medicines will work. We're going to be optimistic, okay?"

"Okay."

Shortly after, my mom and I made a sweatshirt that I could wear when I started going to NIH. It had HIV in great big letters, with "Hugs InVited" spelled out in purple and pink puffy paints. It was my secret spy wear, since I could only wear it at NIH. This was one of the ways we got through the tough stuff; when life deals you crap, just go with it and make a sweatshirt.

We then began our journey into the new world of drug protocols. My first visit to NIH took place around Halloween and my nurse was dressed as Batman. It was very symbolic of my life's journey: far from normal, but never lacking in fun.

While rigorous and tiring, my days at NIH became surprisingly positive experiences. The protocols required that I go to the hospital every 3 months for a battery of tests and procedures. By this time in my life, at the ripe old age of 10, I was pretty accustomed to the medical world, and it didn't faze me much. My NIH visits became bonding rituals with my mom. On NIH mornings, Mom and I began our long day of driving and testing with a stop at McDonalds for orange juice, a hash brown, and a sausage biscuit, hold the biscuit. God bless those little greasy miracles.

When we got to NIH, we parked in the underground garage and took the elevators up to the 13th floor. Then we checked in, got my vital signs taken, and scoped out which doctors and nurses were working that day. I checked out the snack station; they usually had good juice and graham crackers to munch on. My next stop was always the playroom to start a craft or play the Addams Family pinball machine. That was the coolest thing ever—a free pinball machine that I could play as many times as I wanted! Amazing! I made the recreational therapy staff insane because I either played that pinball machine that made an awful racket, or I picked the most complicated crafts to do. Midway through my project, I always got bored and asked, "Could I have another craft?"

"Have you finished that one yet?"

"No, but I'm ready for a new one."

"You have to finish that project before you start on another one."

Every time. It's a good thing they kept everything under lock and key, because I was a manic craft master.

It was always time for labs when I was in the playroom, so the nurse knew where to find me.

"Hey Jamie, I have to steal you away for a few

minutes."

"All right." I knew what was coming, and I knew that I just needed to get it over with.

After my labs, I picked out a prize from the treasure chest and headed back to the playroom.

When the playroom closed, I went back to the waiting room to find my mom and check out the latest news in the Ranger Rick magazine or Highlights. I knew if I sat long enough, the volunteers would come around with the cookie and coffee cart. Free pinball games and free cookies! Come on, this place was pretty awesome.

Soon, the nurse practitioner brought me back for a quick physical, then we headed down to pick up my meds, and we were off. Our first stop out of the hospital was the mall. Rural Pennsylvania did not have good malls, so these became Disneyland to us.

On the busier protocol visits, I had a laundry list of tests and procedures to get through. These would be two-day visits, and we stayed at the Children's Inn on the NIH campus. This was a house for pediatric patients and families to stay when they had multiple days of outpatient tests to get through. For me, it was a funhouse. They had rec rooms, playrooms, TV rooms, computer rooms, a library, and two huge kitchens. When I finished at the clinic, we would go there and explore everything it had to offer. My dad came over after work when we stayed there and we would have epic pool tournaments. He was very skilled at billiards, as he was with most things, but he usually let me win. After countless days at the Children's Inn pool hall/rec room, I actually became pretty good. My dad and I could have gone on the pool hustling circuit like Paul Newman and Tom Cruise.

Back at the clinic, my mom and I became very good at moving swiftly from one department to the next to check off echo, EKG, MRI, CT, chest X ray, occupational therapy, neuropsych testing, and eye exam.

Ech . . . eye exams. Those were the worst. I hated the stingy drops and I could barely stand the photos they sometimes had to take. Brightest lights ever. When they dilated my pupils, my close-up vision became blurrier and blurrier by the second. In the span of 30 minutes, I went from normal Reader's Digest to LARGE PRINT Reader's Digest held at arm's length. Then I was cooked for the rest of the day. My eyes looked huge and black and I couldn't see a thing.

One day I went back to school after one of these appointments because we were having a special assembly. The kids asked me where I had been all day and I told them I had a doctor's appointment. We filed into the all-purpose room and sat down on the floor, waiting for the assembly to begin. The room was buzzing with the noise of hundreds of kids. The teachers sat in metal chairs on the perimeter of the sea of kids.

I was sitting next to boy who looked at me and said, "What's wrong with your eyes? Are you on drugs or something?"

It knocked the wind out of me.

"No, I'm not on drugs! I don't do drugs!"

He turned his attention to something else and I sat there silently, amid the chaos, wondering what had just happened. I was done with my HIV life for the day and was back in school, like the rest of the normal kids. Then this kid asks me if I'm on drugs. Was I caught? Was everyone going to find out about me now? I was so scared that I didn't talk to or look at anyone else for the rest of the day, for fear that my cover would be blown and everyone would find out that I was HIV positive.

I went home that day and cried my little dilated eyes out. I felt different and was ashamed about something I couldn't help. I was so afraid that people would find out about me and that they would hate me.

When I did go back to NIH, at least I could be myself without lying. I felt comfortable there, because I knew I wasn't in jeopardy of being ostracized. Still, while I felt comfortable at NIH, there were a few unhappy memories that left a lasting impression. When starting a drug protocol, patients typically have to undergo an enormous amount of testing to gather baseline information. For this first protocol, I had to get a lumbar puncture. The nurse told me about the procedure and it appropriately freaked me out. Having a needle stuck into my spine was not at all on my list of Top Ten Things I wanted to do that day. But it had to be done.

"We promise that we will only have to do this once, okay?" the nurse practitioner said, trying to reassure me.

My parents taught me that when things have to be

done, the only thing to do is to find a way to get through it. The lumbar puncture (LP) was scheduled for that afternoon, so the coping process began. I had all the information I needed and it was time to find something to look forward to. My parents were always the best at giving me prizes after really crappy stuff like this, so my mom and I talked about what special thing I would like after I get through this. I don't think of this as bribery as much as goal-oriented motivation. Nothing wrong with that.

Like many little girls, I loved all things fluffy and kitten-related, so naturally my first request was a kitten. Aim high, right? My mother, never one to be duped, quickly nixed that one, and suggested other treats that did not involve food, water, and a litter box. Fair enough. She agreed that we could pick something out at the store after we were finished.

It just so happened that this particular day was pincushion day for some reason. That day, I had to get my normal labs drawn and I also had to get five allergy shots. This involved five injections of allergy serums into my forearms. Not fun! We got those two things out of the way in the morning. I walked into the playroom with one sore arm and started on a craft. There were other kids in the playroom too, but I just want to sit by myself and do my crafts.

A few minutes later the nurse practitioner brought me back for my physical. She told me that they were going to give me some medicine right before the LP to help me calm down. We went back to the waiting room. I was a ball of nerves, anxiously anticipating the

LP. Then the nurse practitioner came back again.

Didn't we already do this? I thought.

"Jamie, we have to do one other thing today that we weren't planning for. There was a little boy in the playroom today who may have chickenpox."

"Who is it?" I asked.

"I can't tell you that because it's private."

I was genuinely concerned for this kid. Chickenpox can be deadly for people with HIV, so this was a very serious issue. I felt so bad for him.

"Is he okay?"

"Yes, he'll be just fine."

Whew. Close call.

Okay, well, thanks for telling me, I was thinking. Now let me get back to my Ranger Rick.

"This means that we have to give you two shots to protect you from getting it too."

"What?" I asked, fully upset now. I began to cry. Wasn't this day painful enough? I was trying to focus on getting through the LP, and then they spring this on me?

"I'm sorry, Jamie. I know this stinks."

I hugged my mom and cried. I had had quite enough of this day.

"Sweetie, I know this is hard, but we have to do it. They'll make it fast, okay?" my mom said.

"Okayyyy," I said through slobbery tears. This sucked.

Thus, I got the varicella-zoster immune globulin injection, affectionately known as the VZIG shot, or more affectionately known as the pain in my ass.

Literally. I had to get two shots in my hiney to protect me from developing chickenpox. Now, I've never actually seen a viscosity analysis done on the VZIG serum, but I'm imagining that it would be in the full-sugar maple syrup/caramel sundae sauce category of thickness. This stuff was thick. Better safe than sorry, but OW! I lay face down on the table with my pants down, they counted to three, then POW! One down, one to go. Except this time I knew how much it hurt, so I tensed up even more. One, two, three, POW!

Good grief. I hadn't even gotten to the big procedure and I was exhausted, in pain, and pretty much spent.

I stayed in the treatment room because I was in no mood to socialize, and I needed to take the sedative for my LP. I drank the medicine and sat in the vinyl chair, just waiting. Waiting for the LP. Waiting for the medicine to take effect. Waiting for that wretched day to be over.

The sedative was supposed to calm me down and make me feel free as a bird. Instead, it made me paranoid. I feared the procedure even more, and now I was so looped out that I couldn't even help myself calm down. In essence, the drugs doped up my good coping skills. I sat in that chair in utter fear and panic.

They took me into another procedure room when it was time for the LP. I was panicked and terrified. The room was small, with barely enough room for the nurse practitioner, the equipment, and my mom. I got onto the table and they positioned me for the LP. Ironically, the ideal position is the fetal position, which very much matched how I felt at the time: a defenseless infant with no control. My mom was sitting right in front of me holding my hands and talking me through everything. I was scared and just wanted it to be over. I just had to do this once, and then we would be done, I kept telling myself.

They inserted the needle and it was incredibly painful. I didn't have any numbing medicine on the area, and the sedatives were a joke. I just had to get through it. I was curled up on the table, crying, and just trying to hold still. Finally, the needle came out. My body relaxed and my mom comforted me, telling me that I had done such a great job. I began to feel my favorite emotion in the world—relief. I finally relaxed. Even though I was still sore, it was over.

"Jamie, you did a great job," the nurse practitioner said, "but we have to do it again. Unfortunately, we got some blood in the sample and we can't use it."

I lost it. I was in utter and complete hysterics at this point. I had done my part. I had gotten through it. Only once. They promised. I was devastated. I sobbed hysterically. I honestly didn't know how I was going to get through another one.

My mom, usually my pillar of strength, was visibly upset at this point. She was eye level with me, but she looked up at the nurse practitioner and said, through gritted teeth, "You promised her that you would only have to do it once. You are doing it one more time, and then we are done, whether you get it or not."

"We'll get it."

"Sweetie, we have to do this one more time and then

we are done," she told me.

I couldn't even respond, I was too hysterical.

In a moment of pure motherly love, she said, "You can get a kitten! We'll get you a kitten!" She knew that at this point I was so broken down that I just needed something to bring me up. Through hysterical sobs, I said "Okay" and we hunkered down for one more go. This time hurt even more than the first, since they were going into a spot that was already sore.

Thankfully, the second time was a charm, and they got a usable sample. Good thing for my parents, too, otherwise, they would have been the proud owners of a kitten and a brand new pony that day.

Feeling relief for real this time, I lay on the table, mentally and physically exhausted. I couldn't even move. The staff quietly cleaned up the room, not making eye contact with my mom. She held me close while watching them, willing them to get out before she pounced. We sat quietly in the room until we got the energy together to get up and leave. All I knew was that it was an awful day, and I just wanted to go home.

We closed the books on that terrible day and I set my sights on the light at the end of the tunnel: my new kitten. Now my mom had to figure out how to tell my dad that we were about to adopt another cat. Since we moved to Pennsylvania, we had turned into little cat hoarders. We lived in the woods, and they were all outside cats, so it wasn't THAT big a deal. All it meant was that when we put the food outside, 10 cats came running, instead of the normal two or three. Yes, 10. We were becoming country folk, what did you expect?

Rounding up each cat to take it to the vet was like.... herding cats (oh, that makes sense now). The truth is, we would have adopted anything that showed up on our doorstep, and we pretty much did. Dogs, cats, mountain lions. All were welcome. We had become the Jolie-Pitts of animals.

My dad tried to squelch this animal hoarding movement, but he didn't help the cause much either; he loved them just as much as we did. In fact, he may have been the worst offender. One day he came home with a baby deer in his car. A baby deer. We saw him walk up the sidewalk with the fawn in his arms, and ran to the door. Noticing the ruckus, my mom headed over to the door too. We were all on our front porch, fawning over this . . . fawn (oh, that makes sense now). Heather and I tried to pet him. My dog sniffed at him, thinking, what kind of dog are you, weirdo?

"What. Is. That?" my mom said to my dad. We all knew that look. It was the 'are you out of your mind?' look. We just quietly stroked the deer.

"It was abandoned on the side of the road. It was trying to get over the stone wall, and it kept falling down. Its mother had left it behind," he explained.

"Put. It. Back."

"Oh, it's okay. I just wanted to girls to see it. I'll take him back in a little bit."

"Mmmm hmmmmm...."

Sadly, we didn't get to keep the deer. My dad set it free, and it probably became a social outcast in the deer world, having come home smelling like kids and dogs.

So it wasn't that uncommon for our family to

accumulate assorted pets. A few days after the disastrous LP, my mom took me to the SPCA to pick out my kitten. I could barely contain myself as we pulled up to the drab-looking building. We walked inside and heard a cacophony of meowing.

We were led into a room that had a caged-off section of kittens and cats. As we walked up to the cage, some of the cats went crazy and started climbing up the wire door. I looked at an adorable gray and black tabby cat who was scaling the wall.

"He's cute," I said.

"He is cute. But he's a little hyper. Look at those cute ones. The ones that are sitting down."

I looked over and saw a tiny black kitten sitting on a plank of wood. She was just sitting there, amidst all the wild cats running all over the place. I took one look at her and fell in love.

"I like that one," I said as I pointed her out to my mom.

They brought her out to me and she snuggled right into my arms. She purred as I pet her tiny little head. I didn't even have to think about it—she was perfect, and I knew she was my pick. I didn't put her down until we got her home.

I named her Bun Bun LP MD. Bun Bun for the shots in the butt, LP for the . . . LP, duh, and MD, because she had to have medical credentials. She was the best cat ever.

CHAPTER FIVE

I was now a secret agent. A kid with a secret I was allowed to keep. Having been raised with solid moral values, the concept of strategic dishonesty was new to me, but I got pretty good at it. When anyone asked why I went to the hospital, missed school, or took medicines, I said, "because I have a problem with my heart." Technically not a lie, so I was still good. It was better to fudge the truth than to risk being socially ostracized, possibly kicked out of elementary school, and shunned by the community.

As I got used to living this secret life with HIV, I came to expect a certain level of ignorance and prejudice from many people. The world just wasn't yet educated on what HIV was and what it wasn't. The general population wasn't convinced that you couldn't catch it from a sneeze, or that HIV positive people weren't all gay men. I understood this reality, even at a young age, and I knew that was why I had to keep it a secret. However, I also knew that there were people who were supposed to understand and were supposed to be supportive. Apparently I overestimated some people in the medical community, as I would soon find out.

The ever-popular eye exam came to be a very interesting part of my NIH visits. Not only did I hate getting the stinging drops that make me look like a drug addict, as I learned from assembly day, but one particular physician was an added bonus. During a protocol visit, I sat in the chair, eyes dilated and blurry, waiting for the doctor to come in. Finally, in walked Dr. Personality. Barely even looking at me or my mother, he walked over to my chart and sat down to review it. It is an impressive thing, thicker than most encyclopedias and surely capable of breaking a toe if it were dropped on one's foot. In all its glorious magnitude, however, it only took once glance at the first page to see: "Primary Diagnosis: HIV positive."

Ding ding ding! ALERT! ALERT! ALERT!! It was as if he had just entered a hazmat situation. His demeanor went from cold to icy-frozen-popsicle, and he immediately put on gloves and a mask. My mom and I looked at each other as if to say, Is this guy for real? Didn't every doctor know that you couldn't get it by touching someone? Well, apparently, he missed that day of eye doctor school. He proceeded to examine my eyes in his protective gear. I got through the exam quietly, following his instructions: "look up, look down, look straight ahead" (into my blinding light of lunacy). His gear effectively protected him from my magical strain of HIV that could jump person-to-person through the air, and from all hopes of logical thinking.

We later found out that this particular doctor was notorious for his overzealous protective garb, thereby making most of us HIV kids feel like little petri dishes of disease. One mom told us that this guy wore a full-on protective suit during her 6-year-old son's eye exam. This poor child was terrified when he walked in looking like the government guys from ET. His mom swiftly intervened and said, "Look, sweetie, he dressed up for you for Halloween!" Moms can be so great.

I learned not to take things like this personally, because it would only make me mad. Sadly, even people who should know better sometimes don't.

My family quickly learned that we had to be very careful of who we told about my HIV status. In fact, our best bet was to tell as few people as possible. This was still the time when people wouldn't touch you if you had AIDS. Children and families were uprooted from their communities and homes because of pure, unfounded fear. Thus, we only told immediate family members, school nurses, my pediatrician, and a select group of family friends.

Since moving to Pennsylvania, we kept in touch with our friends who lived down the street from us in Maryland. I missed hanging out with my best friend Tessa, and I wanted her to visit me in our new house.

"Mom, can we set up a sleepover with Tessa?"

"Sure, Sweetie. I'll talk to her mom and see what we can set up."

I was so excited!

A few weeks passed, and my mom hadn't said

anything to me about a sleepover. I figured it was just because our families' schedules were busy, so I asked again.

"Mom, when am I going to have a sleepover with Tessa?"

"I don't know if we're going to able to set that up," she said, and quickly changed the subject.

A few more weeks passed, and I was getting antsy. All I wanted to do was hang out with my friend! Why was that so hard? I tried one more time. "Mom, I really want to see Tessa. When can she come over?"

My mom sighed. "Sweetie, Tessa isn't going to come over at all. We told her parents about your HIV, and they don't want her to come over."

"Why not?"

"They just don't know all the facts about how it's spread."

"But her dad is a doctor! How come he doesn't know?"

"I know. Even doctors don't know everything, Sweetie. They just don't understand."

I was devastated. How could they take my friend away from me just because they didn't understand? And her dad was a doctor—shouldn't he have known better? I always knew that my HIV status might keep strangers away from me, strangers who just didn't know any better, but I never thought it would take away my best friend. I never saw her again after that. I said goodbye, from afar, to my best friend, with the stark realization that sometimes, this thing I had was more powerful than I was.

This harsh reality quickly opened my eyes to how dangerous it could be to tell the wrong person about my HIV status. Who knows what people might do to me if they thought I could put them in harm's way? So I continued living my double life: one as a normal kid, and one who was HIV positive.

I fell into a comfortable pattern of living this double life. At NIH, I was a kid with HIV, like the other kids with me in the waiting room. Everyone knew, and no one made a big deal about it. At school, I was a "normal" kid who loved caboodles and New Kids on the Block. In the back of my mind, though, I always wondered what it would be like to tell my friends the truth. I don't remember people even saying HIV aloud in my rural hometown. It was assumed that things like HIV didn't happen to people in small towns who led simple, peaceful lives. While I desperately wanted to tell my friends who I really was, fear kept me quiet. Fear of being outcast, harassed, or even hurt. I didn't know what people would do if they knew, and I wasn't about to find out.

As a child, I wrote about this, as writing was one of the safe ways I could express myself. This was incredibly therapeutic for me, allowing me to get my little secret world out, even if it was only on paper.

At age 11, I wrote:

Sometimes I want to tell people about my virus, but then I think about the Pros and Cons. Some Pros that I think about are that I wouldn't have to hide anything or lie to anyone. I feel bad about lying, but then again, I can't tell anyone. I like coming to NIH because I can say it without having to worry about the way that people will take it.

But then there're always the Cons. People could just forget about the facts and just get away from me. They could tell their parents, but then the parents would maybe want them to get out of the school, but from my point of view, they have nothing to worry about. Another Con would be that the people that I tell and that I trust to keep it a secret could tell someone else and then they would tell everyone else so then everyone would get away from me. Even if I tell them and they know the facts, they just wouldn't understand. Then there are always the people who wouldn't believe me or the facts.

Obviously, the cons outweighed the pros for me, and I kept my life a secret. I was able to open up to my family, my friends at NIH, and my journal. This kept me going and helped get me through the secrets and the hiding. When I was frustrated, I wrote about it. When I had something to say to other people, I wrote about it. When I just couldn't tell anyone, I wrote about it.

Still, a part of me always wondered what it would be like to be open about being HIV positive. I had a lot to tell people, but I had to keep it contained. When I was 12, I decided that I needed to tell the world, in my own secret way, what I thought they should know about HIV:

I would like the world to know how it is to have

HIV. Some people think that people who have HIV or AIDS are weird. If only they would realize what it is like and what you have to go through. I think that if you took a survey to see how regular people react to the situation (knowing someone with HIV), you would get some very negative results. I would like the world to know that you are just as normal as the next person even if you have HIV or AIDS. I would like the world to know that you cannot get the virus just from standing in the same room as someone with it, or hugging someone, or touching the same countertop, or even using the same cup or dish or utensils. The people who criticize them don't have any idea what HIV and AIDS people go through. And what they really don't know is that we need their support and love, not their jokes and insensitivity. The truth is that having HIV and AIDS is scary and it won't just go away. It is with you when you go to sleep, when you wake up, when you go to school, and all other times. But there are some good things about having HIV and AIDS. Almost everyone you meet has a happy face on. You meet new friends at the clinic and they understand, so it is a great place to be!!!

Man, I had a lot of feelings to get out. I was turning into a little journalist, like Carrie Bradshaw with an entirely different subject matter. This is what kept me sane, though. I couldn't tell anyone my secret and I was way too old to have an imaginary friend, so I poured my secret life out on the pages. This was how I dealt with the isolation, the frustration, the reality of my secret life.

I continued to process this in my writing, and as a teenager I wrote:

> "Whether or not to tell your friends about your HIV Diagnosis"
>
> First, you need to know whether you can really trust the friend you are planning to tell. If you think this friend will not be able to keep it a secret, FORGET IT and pick another friend. Just because the person is your best friend does not mean they will be able to keep it a secret.
>
> Second, remember to be sure about who you are telling. Be prepared for people who do not understand, like your friends' parents. Once you do tell, try and go on with your life. There will always be people who do not understand and who may stay away from you. The important thing is that you keep your true friends. The others were never really true friends.
>
> Third, once you do tell, don't lie again. You're finally out of that web of lies and make new friends who will be true friends.

It seems that I was writing a handbook for people with HIV. I was writing to a virtual audience, because I couldn't talk to my actual friends. It was my world on paper. In another writing session at age 14, I wrote:

> This virus can drive you crazy! If affects me in

a lot of different ways. One way is that I have to take disgusting medicine. And at very inconvenient times. Sometimes I feel tired, but some days I feel great. Sometimes my counts go up and sometimes they go down. The virus just can't make up its mind on whether it will be nice or not. I think about it a lot, and sometimes it scares me a lot, but my mom or dad is always there to help me. Most kids my age never think about dying. Most kids my age never think about that and they really take life for granted, but this has helped me understand that every little day means a lot to my family and I, just that we're together. I think that this virus has not only made me sick and sad, but it's also made me a lot happier because I cherish each day with my family.

A lot of people have conflicting feelings on this matter, and some of them are not very good, but if you are always positive (no joke intended) you will do alright! You've just got to keep things in perspective. I know a lot of you have the same feelings, and I just hope that this will help you understand that you're not in it alone.

I processed all of this at a young age, and it helped me live my double life without going crazy. My HIV- and non-HIV selves were becoming fairly well distinguished. My HIV self began making friends with the "regulars" at NIH. These were kids I met in the playroom, did an occasional craft with, and sat next to in the treatment room for blood draws—you know, the usual kid stuff. It was sort of like a bridge club for sick kids. Our parents would catch up over the free coffee from the roaming coffee cart, and we kids would just shoot the breeze. One day I met a boy named Justin. He was a little younger than me and he was HIV positive too. He had a big sister about the age of my older sister, Heather. Our moms hit it off, and soon we were not only clinic buddies, but also best friends. We were at the age where boys and girls weren't supposed to like hanging out together, because you could catch cooties. Well, I guess one could say that we both already had cooties, so it was all good.

My mom and Justin's mom planned our clinic days together so we could see each other. We met in the playroom and palled around all day together. Justin didn't know that he was HIV positive, and he had a harder time dealing with everything. He hated getting his blood drawn, but I tried to help him through it. When it was time to go back to the treatment room he got upset, so we walked back together. I sat next him as he cried quiet sad tears in the treatment room chair. I held his hand and he squeezed mine the whole time until the needle came out, at which point he looked at me and smiled with pride. He always bounced back just like that. We picked out prizes from the treasure box and got back to the business of hanging out in the playroom.

Our parents often made arrangements for play dates together; we only lived an hour or so away from each other. We both loved video games and playing around on his swing set. Justin decided to get a mega-video game system for his Make-A-Wish. He was so excited, and shortly after he got it, we made a trip to his house to see it. It was like a Nintendo shrine. It covered practically the whole wall of his den. We played that thing until our eyes were crossed. We had so much fun—we never talked about the hospital or HIV. My mom told me that I couldn't talk about HIV around him since he didn't know his status, which was fine by me. It never came up anyway; all we cared about was having fun and being kids.

We were two peas in a pod, Justin and me. One day our parents planned a sleepover for after our clinic visits. We were so excited to finish up at the clinic and hop in our car for a weekend of fun. In my mom's car on the way to our house, Justin quickly leaned over and kissed my cheek. I looked over at him, and he was beaming, saying, "I did it!" He was so cute. I remember thinking, Eww, a boy just kissed me! but being touched nonetheless. He looked at me with a *Ha! I just kissed you!* look, and I looked at him with a *Goober! Why'd you just kiss me?* look. Then we promptly resumed our normal relationship of just being friends.

We spent the weekend running through the woods and climbing all over the big boulders by my creek. When it came time to take our medicine, we didn't have to hide it from each other. It was no big deal. At the end of the weekend, his mom picked him up with the promise that we would see each other again soon.

A few months later, my mom and I were at home and the phone rang. She answered, and went into her bedroom to take the call. I was in our living room reading a book. After a few minutes, my mom walked out of her bedroom and sat down next to me on the couch.

"Sweetie," she said, "there's something I need to tell you."

I put my book down and looked at her. What could it be this time? I had pretty much had it with these conversations. I knew this tone and I knew it wasn't good.

"Honey, Justin died."

"What?"

"Justin died Sweetie."

"But he wasn't even sick. He was fine."

"I know. The last time you saw him, he wasn't sick. But since then, he began to get very sick and his little body gave out on him."

There were no more words at this point, only tears. I curled up in my mom's arms and cried. My mom cried with me. "I'm so sorry," she said.

I cried.

I didn't know what to do or what to think. Justin and I had the same thing, and he died. Why was I so healthy, while he was getting sick and dying? Was it going to be that fast for me?

I wasn't ready for this. I had processed through my own mortality at this young age, but I wasn't prepared to lose my friends. I knew there was a chance I would die, but I didn't think it would ever happen to my friends. I wasn't expecting to be one of the people left behind.

At school, I couldn't tell my classmates or my

teachers that one of my best friends had just died. I kept it inside and tried to be normal and stay under the radar. A few days later, my mom asked if I wanted to go to Justin's funeral.

"They are going to have it in a couple of days. Do you think you would like to go to it?"

"I don't know. Is his coffin going to be open?"

"Yes, I think it will."

"I don't know if I want to go."

"That's fine Sweetie. We don't have to go."

In the end I couldn't do it. I couldn't see him in any way other than my smiling and carefree friend. Instead of going to his funeral, my mom and I planned our own ceremony for Justin. I picked out a red Japanese maple at the garden center, and my dad planted it in our front yard on the day of his funeral. We also got a yellow smiley face balloon from a party store and released it in the parking lot; not a very poignant setting, but it was still perfect. As we drove home from the parking lot, we were listening to the radio, just taking it all in. *Can You Feel the Love Tonight* from *The Lion King* came on the radio. As I listened to this song, Justin became very close to me again.

It's enough for this wide-eyed wanderer that we got this far.

And it was enough. I realized that even though Justin's life was too short, he soaked up every minute of it. He went through pain, but he always bounced back with a smile on his face. He was a wide-eyed wanderer, up against something too big for him to beat, but still just being a kid and having fun. This is how

Justin stays in my memory.

When Justin died, I was reminded of how serious this was. I had the same thing that my friend just died from. I was healthy now, but how long would that last? Would I live long enough to go to the prom? Would I graduate high school? Of course no one knew the answer to that. We just carried on with life, trying to keep me as healthy as possible.

I had to depend on other people to stay healthy, too. I was at the mercy of scientific research to keep developing new medications. In order for that to happen, people had to think that AIDS was a problem. I mistakenly thought that everyone knew this. If people are sick, you want to make them better. Especially kids. No one would have wanted Justin to die. Everyone cared about keeping the rest of us alive. Right?

I soon learned that I gravely overestimated some people. I was 14 at the time, and it was winter—a typical cold and snowy Pennsylvania winter. I was snuggled inside with hot chocolate and a Newsweek, one of my go-to favorites from years spent in waiting rooms.

I was reading the "Perspectives" section, and I came across the following:

> "The problem with AIDS is: you got it, you die. So why are we spending money on the issue?" – Lt. Gov. R.

I read that quote and felt like I had been sucker

punched in the face. It came out of left field and it hurt like hell. I was completely unprepared to deal with such blatant hatred. It was as if this man was looking into my eyes and saying, "I don't care if you die, Jamie." Worse yet, one of my best friends had just died, so this person was, in essence, saying that he didn't care that Justin died. That his life was inconsequential, as was mine.

I couldn't fight this fight on my own, and ignorance like this meant that people weren't fighting for me to live. This told me that it was possible for people to turn their back on me. There were people out there who didn't care if I died.

This struck me to the core and broke me down. When I read it, I started weeping. Until then, I had never been so hurt by someone's words. In fact, I didn't think it was possible for someone to be so hurtful—and a leader, no less. I thought they were supposed to hold babies and say cheese? This wasn't supposed to happen, this kind of surprise attack. I was supposed to be aware of when I might encounter stupidity and negativity; I was supposed to be able to prepare myself. But I wasn't, and I couldn't. I was raw and defenseless. A child, broken down by the words of a cold man. I was angry. I was shocked. I was scared. What if more people felt like this? What if people read his quote and thought, *You know, he's right; why ARE we spending money on this?* What if people stopped researching HIV drugs? My life literally depended on that, and I was well aware of that fact. If everyone felt like he did, what would happen to me? I felt as if he was telling the world to leave me out to die.

I ran to my mom and just cried in her arms. I was overwhelmed by how much this hurt me. It reminded me that even though I was surrounded by such positive people, there was a cruel world out there that was capable of hurting me tremendously. As always, my mom knew just what to do and say. She comforted me and told me that his quote was published so that people could see how foolish and asinine he was. She assured me that he was getting this attention because it was an absurd thing to say, and that most people reading it would think that he was a monster. It eased my mind to be reminded that most people weren't this cruel. Still, I had to speak my own mind in response to his terrible comment. When my tears stopped, I got to writing, and composed this letter to him:

Dear Lt. Gov. R.,

You probably don't receive very many letters from a 14-year-old who is concerned about the comments that a politician makes to reporters. I happened to have read a statement you made, quoted in Newsweek's "Perspectives" (1/17/1994). The quote read: "The problem with AIDS is: you got it, you die. So why are we spending money on the issue?"

Allow me to introduce myself. My name is Jamie and I was infected with HIV (that's the virus that causes AIDS) in 1982 through contaminated blood that was used during open heart surgery. I have been living with HIV for at least 11 years. Let me tell you what it is like. It is frightening, scary, sometimes lonely, challenging, and frustrating. Frightening because you never know when your last birthday will be. Scary because of all of the blood tests and IVs that you have to have. Lonely because lots of times, you just feel that you don't have any real friends at school who you can relate to. Plus you never know how people will react to you or your family if you tell them the truth about what you're living with. Challenging because you have to meet each day with courage, confidence, and faith. Frustrating because many groups are working so hard to raise money to end this horrific disease and when you finally feel that our society has made some progress towards accepting people with AIDS, comments like yours show up in Newsweek and other public places.

Your comment devastated me. It devastated my family. And I'm sure that it devastated many other people who know, care about, or live with this disease. I can't remember a time when just a simple comment made me cry so much. It made me so angry that I decided to write you this letter. I believe that I am writing this on behalf of tens of thousands of people who feel the same way. I sure hope that you will never need to learn firsthand what living with HIV is all about. I hope AIDS never attacks anyone you love or care about. I believe that if it did, your attitude would change. In the meantime, for us, every dollar used towards medical research brings hope that we are a little closer to finding a cure.

Please reconsider your statement, now knowing that there are people out there who really need everyone's support. I choose to believe that every human life has value; that we as a society have no "disposable people." Every positive comment brings us a step closer towards living a normal life. Every negative comment, like the one that you made, throws us many years backwards and unnecessarily reminds us that we are a little different.

With hope that this will make a difference,
Jamie

I never heard back from him. I don't know if he ever read it, and if he did, if it made a difference; I can only hope that it did. It took a while to recover from that one. Once I did, though, I realized that yes, I would encounter small-minded people with hurtful words, and yes, they are often the first ones to spout off their opinions for the world to hear. More importantly, though, I would encounter resilience and strength from the people in my corner. Luckily, the people in my corner outnumbered the idiots.

CHAPTER SIX

MY life changed again when I was 12 years old, in the back woods of Connecticut. Nestled there, behind an inconspicuous wooden sign, lies The Hole in the Wall Gang Camp (THITWGC), a safe haven for children with serious and rare diseases. It was founded in 1988 by Paul Newman, a man who would change my life forever. "Hole in the Wall" is named for the secret place that no one knew about in Butch Cassidy and the Sundance Kid. Most people probably never even notice the camp as they drive by. What they don't know is that this place is pure magic.

Initially I was not a fan of the idea of summer camp. First of all, it involves camping, and we all know how I feel about that. No thank you. I think camping is an insult to the inventors of plumbing and electricity. No really, I applaud people who can rough it in the great outdoors just for fun—I'm just not one of those people.

So that was strike one against the idea of summer camp. Strike two was that it was in Connecticut. The thought of leaving my routine—my home, my meds, my hospital—was one thing, but leaving it seven hours away was quite another. Okay, honestly, how crazy did I make my parents that they wanted to ship me off to Connecticut for 10 days? Strike three was that I didn't know anyone there. The idea was just plain scary. Strike four, the big one, was that I was afraid that my meds would get messed up if my mom wasn't there to give them to me.

Therefore, when my mom brought up the idea of going to this "great camp in Connecticut where they have people there to give you your meds," I said, "thanks but no thanks." Moving on. If I wanted to go camping, I would throw a sleeping bag on my living room floor and make s'mores in the microwave. And even then, I probably wouldn't make it through the night before crawling into my cozy bed.

Despite my initial refusal, my mom and dad knew that this would be so good for me, so they tried again to convince me that I should go. They even had a camp counselor, Karen, call me to tell me what they did there, and how cool it was. I asked questions about what kind of activities they had, and she told me about some of them. I still wasn't sold until she said, "Do you know what else we have here?"

"What?"

"Horses."

ZOINKS! This got my attention. Like most little girls, I was obsessed with horses, and had always begged my parents to get one. (I got a kitten that one time, so I figured I would keep shooting for the moon.)

"Can I ride them?" I asked.

"You can! You can ride them every day if you want!" Karen said.

Are you kidding me? This was my dream. I could ride horses every day for 10 days? Stick a fork in me and call me done. They could send me to Argentina, and I would gladly go for the joy of riding horses every day.

Wooed by the promise of horses, I caved in and finally agreed to go to Hole in the Wall. But I was still terrified. My mom and I packed my bags with everything on the list of things to bring. We piled the family into the car for the seven-hour drive to Connecticut and were on our way. That car ride was nerve-wracking. I tried to sleep as much as I could to escape the anxiety, but nothing helped.

We finally arrived in the little town of Ashford and decided to stop for pizza right before we arrived at camp. I was a ball of nerves. We sat at a booth and ate our pizza, and I was just a wound up little nutcase. I don't remember ever being that nervous in my life, which is pretty remarkable considering what my life had been like until that point.

After lunch we continued on for another four miles until we found the entrance to camp. On this particular day, it wasn't hard to miss at all. Under the wooden "The Hole in the Wall Gang Camp" sign were a bunch of yahoos dressed up in costumes: clowns, huge cowboy hats, ridiculous outfits. When we turn left into the driveway, they all went crazy, screaming and hollering, "Welcome to camp!!!!! What's your name?"

Wide-eyed and bewildered, I replied quietly, "Jamie," at which point they all screamed, "Jamie is here! Woo-hoooo!!" I smiled, and promptly rolled up my window.

I was still cautious, but overall pretty thrilled that they were so excited that I was there. We continued driving up the dirt road into camp and I looked around in amazement. To the left was a magnificent lake, banked by a campsite on the opposite side, and a huge boathouse directly across. The dirt road rounded a bend, where it was flanked by great big boulders. We were passing through the Hole in the Wall and entering a magical safe haven.

We pulled up to the registration area and saw more excited counselors and elated kids. It was organized chaos, and I was already beginning to feel the magic of this place. I was still shy and nervous, but I liked what I saw. We checked in, got name tags ("Hello, My Name is....Terrified") and they unloaded my bags onto a big truck. Next, my parents and I hopped on a golf cart and a counselor drove us down to the main camp area. I still held on to my mom and dad for dear life, but cautiously looked around as we drove. We rounded the bend that brought us to the main area of camp and we were all stupefied. This. Place. Was. Disneyland— but a million times better, as I would soon find out. The cabins were enormous and the buildings were all laid out like a western town—they had everything: a woodshop, arts and crafts, a huge dining hall, a two-story gym, an Olympic-sized pool, ropes courses, a massive theater building, the lake, and a boathouse.

We drove into the center of camp and I looked around in amazement. We rounded the bend, and I nearly wet my pants at what I saw next, the piece de resistance. Right there, before my very eyes, were the horses. There really were horses there; they weren't just saying that to woo me! I squeezed my parents' arms with a quiet little squeal of excitement.

"Oh my gosh, Jamie, there are those horses you've been waiting to see!" my mom said. She turned to the counselor and said, "She was so nervous to come here and it wasn't until they told her about the horses that she agreed to come."

"Well then let's go see them!" the counselor said.

All smiles, they took me over to see them. I walked up to a black and white horse, held by another counselor named Leslie.

"Hi there," Leslie said.

"Hi," I said, my eyes fixed on the horse.

"You can come over and pet him."

My parents knew that I was sold at this point, and smiled as I walked over to meet the horse.

"Do you want to ride him?" Leslie asked.

I looked back at my parents, and they both nodded their approval. I looked back at Leslie and nodded with a big smile. I put on my helmet, got up on the horse, and Leslie took me for a ride around the woods.

"Is this your first time at camp?" she asked.

"Yes."

"Oh, you are going to love it. Are you excited?"

"Yes. I'm going to have my birthday here."

"That's so exciting! What day is it?"

"It's on the 9th."

She turned around and said to me, "That's my birthday too."

I was so thrilled—I had a new friend and a birthday buddy. This place was going to be all right.

After the horse ride, our next stop was at the infirmary to check in all of my medications. Okay, here's where we get down to business. Everybody, pay attention, I was thinking, we have a lot of stuff to cover. Well, as it turns out, the full staff of nurses and physicians at camp pretty much has their stuff together. With hundreds of medically-fragile kids passing through their gates every summer, they could deal with almost any medical issue without blinking an eye. I was actually a cake walk for them. HIV meds? No problem. Well then. I guess I'm not as complicated as I thought I was. Relieved that all was kosher with my meds, we moved on to the cabins.

Fifteen cabins were divided into five units of three cabins each. Every unit had a color, and every cabin had a number. I was a Yellow 4 kid. My bags were waiting in my cabin, and I joined more counselors and a few other kids who had already arrived. I walked in with my parents to a huge room with ten beds. I looked around for an available bed, but all of them had bags on them already. Oh no, I thought, they forgot to add me to the list! They don't have any room for me. We drove all this way, and now we're going to have to go stay at the Holiday Inn, which, I'm pretty sure, doesn't offer pony rides! I knew this was a bad idea....

I looked at my parents and said, "I don't see any free beds. They all have bags on them," and my new counselor Karen said, "Oh no, those bags are for you! Just pick a bed that doesn't have anyone else's stuff on it."

Oh thank God.

There was room for me after all, and I got a bag full of goodies? Nice! I claimed a top bunk in the corner and started to go through my bag of treasures.

Once I was all settled in, it was time to say goodbye to my parents. I think they had been dreading this moment for weeks. They feared I would be a hot mess, sobbing, wrapped around their legs, screaming, "don't leave me here, you cruel, cruel people!"

Well, that shy, terrified little kid from 60 minutes ago was long gone. I think I said something like, "'K, bye, see ya!" while giving them a half-assed hug and running back into the cabin to unpack and start some crafts in the common room.

They were fairly dumbfounded. They were glad I wasn't terrified, but I think they would have appreciated a little sadness at their departure—maybe just a single tear? Yeah, no. I was already immersed in the magic of camp.

To say that camp is amazing would be an understatement, and to try to describe every detail of it wouldn't come close to doing it justice. However, there are a few defining moments that illustrate how this place changed my life.

This was the first time in my life that I ever told

someone I had just met that I was HIV positive. What was amazing was that I did so without any fear of how they would react. I knew I was safe there. For once in my life, my two selves could be joined into one. I could be the normal kid who also happens to have HIV, and I didn't have to differentiate between these two identities. What's more, my HIV status didn't keep me from doing anything that the other kids were doing. This was a place where anything was possible, and illnesses didn't hold anyone back.

Each afternoon, the campers got to pick an activity to do. I discovered that in addition to the horses, I loved fishing. Thus, every day, if I wasn't at the horse barn I was at the boathouse. I bonded quickly with a counselor, Jaysea, and we became the dynamic duo of the open seas. Well, the lake at least. Each afternoon, we gathered our fishing supplies, oars, and life vests, and piled into a rowboat. That lake was the most densely stocked lake on the entire east coast, and I reeled in countless fish, one right after the other. I reeled them in and Jaysea took them off the hook. We did this for a couple of hours every day, and by the end of the session, my fish count was up to 75. I was the Fish Master.

From morning until bedtime, we filled our days with activities. I made about a million crafts: tie-dye shirts, jewelry, decoupage, you name it. I perfected the art of wood burning, and made several plaques at the woodshop. Though the action-packed days should have tired us all out, my cabin mates and I barely slept at night, much to the dismay of the counselors. We even managed to squeeze in polar bear activities, special activities before breakfast, AKA the bane of the counselors' existence. But nothing could stop us. Whether it was running around like a maniac, or lying in the field, staring at the stars in the sky, I had never had so much fun, day in and day out.

The days passed too quickly, and my birthday got closer. At breakfast on my birthday, we walked into the dining hall and our cabin's table was all set up with party decorations. When we got back to the cabin after our morning activity, I walked over to my bed and saw that it was decorated with candy that spelled out "Happy Birthday". After lunch, during rest hour, I got extra time to ride the horses! And to top it all off, the entire camp sang happy birthday to Leslie and me at dinner as we rode around the dining hall in the Birthday Chair that was carried around by all the male counselors. It was embarrassing, but in the best possible way. It made me feel like a queen. It turned out to be the best birthday I ever had, and I'd had some pretty kick ass birthday pool parties growing up. But this took the cake. Never before had I ever felt this special.

That's what this place does, whether it's your birthday or not; people shower you with so much love that you can deal with whatever life gives you to deal with that much easier.

One day, near the end of the session, Paul Newman showed up. He walked into the dining hall quietly. No one made a big deal about the fact that an Oscar-winning celebrity was in our presence, and he wouldn't have wanted it any other way. His passion was seeing the campers live every second of their lives to the fullest while they were at camp. I was excited to meet him, because he was the first movie star I had ever met.

"Is that Paul Newman?" I asked Karen, my counselor.

"Yeah."

"Oh my God. That's so awesome. He's a movie star!"

She laughed. "He's so nice. Do you want to meet him?"

"Yes!"

We were all filing out of the dining hall at the time, and Karen brought me over to meet him.

"Hi," I said, shyly.

"Hi!" he said. "What's your name?"

"Jamie."

"Are you having fun Jamie?"

"Yes. It was my birthday yesterday."

"Happy birthday!"

"Thanks. Can I get a picture with you?"

"Sure!"

That picture of us together is one of my favorites in the world. I'm decked out in about five hand-crafted buttons and five necklaces, with Paul, a man who changed my life forever.

I filled those 10 days of camp with a lifetime of memories. I lived and loved and played like never before. I met the most incredible people in the world. I had the most amazing experiences. My life had truly changed in a way I never thought possible. I didn't want it to end. As the last day of camp drew near, the pit in my stomach grew bigger. How could I leave all this? This, a place I had approached with trepidation and angst, was now my second home.

On pick-up day, I was so hoping that my parents would be late—or better yet, forget about me altogether—so that I could have more precious moments of camp. They, of course, planned to be there right on time to collect me and bring me home. They were probably expecting a tearful reunion with hugs, where I hopped in the car saying, "I missed you guys! Let's go home!"

Sadly for them, this is not what happened. I love my parents dearly, but at that moment, I wanted nothing to do with them. So naturally, I did what any sweet little innocent 13-year-old girl would do.

I hid.

The longer I could evade them, the longer I could stay at camp. Unluckily for me, the counselors were very good at keeping track of where their kids were. Sort of a job requirement, I suppose. My secret spot behind the rock lasted for about 5 minutes, and when I finally saw my parents, ready to take me home, I burst into tears.

My poor parents. All they were trying to do was to give me this great experience, and how do I repay them? With an embarrassing scene. Hysterics. Drama. And a car-full of about 127 camp crafts.

I dragged out my goodbyes as long as I possibly could, hugging, crying, exchanging addresses and vowing to keep in touch. Those friendships would last a lifetime. The people I met that first year of camp, and each year to follow, will always be dear to me.

From that summer on I never spent a birthday at home because I was always at camp. I went back for three more years as a camper, two years as a Leader in Training, two years as a counselor, and my last year as a Unit Leader. Camp truly had become my second home. My years as a counselor were just as amazing as those as a camper. I got to play with hundreds of kids and help them be kids for those few days. I filled my life with camp as much as I possibly could. My family made the seven-hour drive in the off seasons to attend reunion weekends, parties, and my all-time favorite: the Galas.

Every fall, Paul Newman and his show-biz friends organized a variety show—The Gala—to raise money for camp. In my second summer there, I sang "Can You Feel the Love Tonight" at Stage Night, in honor of my friend Justin. It was also the first time I had ever sung by myself in front of a group of people. After that summer, I got a phone call from camp asking if I would be interested in performing at their annual Gala, with a bunch of famous people and a handful of other campers. Ummmm, yes please! They wanted me to play the lead in Snow White. They wanted me, a (previously) shy little kid from Pennsylvania, to come act with all of these famous people. Did they think I was someone else? Seriously, who gets to do this kind of stuff? I quickly said yes before they could come to their senses, and got to work rehearsing my songs. The show was put together by the collective talents of Paul, writer A. E. Hotchner, and composer Cy Coleman. Pat Birch, the renowned choreographer of the film and stage productions of *Grease* and countless others, was the choreographer. No pressure.

In two days of rehearsals I tried to focus on perfecting my role while not getting distracted by Joan Rivers as the narrator, Melanie Griffith and Ann Reinking as the co-evil queens, and Paul Newman, James Naughton, and friends, as the seven dwarves. Again, no pressure. As it turned out, this group of esteemed actors and show biz bigwigs also happened to be amazing people who were sweet and kind. Of course they were; they were devoting their free time to this grand production for charity.

The show went off without a hitch. We performed skit after skit of tongue-in-cheek comedy, with Snow White as our main act, before a packed house. We all had a blast and went out for pizza after the grand finale. By now, the little town of Ashford was accustomed to the invasion of famous folk at this time of year. Exhausted and elated, we crammed ourselves into the little restaurant and celebrated our successful night.

Ms. Birch was talking to my parents after the show in the pizza place. "Jamie did a really good job," she told them.

"Thank you. We think she's fantastic. She has always had a beautiful voice."

"Where do you guys live?"

"Gettysburg, Pennsylvania."

"How far is that to New York City?" she asked.

"It's a hike. Several hours."

"That's too bad. She'd be good."

Come on, parents! This is where they were supposed to say We'd love to move to the city! Do you think we could get front row seats to all of the Broadway shows that she stars in? Which borough is the best for a 14-year-old?

But alas, my parents weren't keen to uproot me to the big city quite yet.

This marked the first of many Galas to come. Every October, I counted down the days until Gala time. The following year I got to play Wendy in Peter Pan, alongside Marisa Tomei (Peter Pan), Glenn Close (narrator), and Paul as drunk Tinkerbell. Yes, Paul Newman as drunk Tinkerbell. Those shows were not for the faint of heart. The writing is meant to appeal to an adult audience, and let's just say it's a good thing we campers didn't understand what we were singing about. It was the first and only time I would see Paul stagger on stage with a beer bottle hanging out of his mouth, in a pink tutu, as drunk Tinkerbell. It was magnificent.

Those Galas were the icing on top of my camp experience. My years were measured by a countdown to camp and Galas. I was on top of the world when I was there, and when I came home, I tucked it away. I couldn't tell anyone about it. It's like that joke where a priest skips church on a Sunday to go golfing. He plays a perfect round of golf, getting one hole-in-one after another. The guilt got to him and he wondered why he had such luck on the day he was skipping his Godly duties. "God," he said, "thank you for this amazing round of golf, but I have to ask. Why did you allow me to have such a perfect game?" "Because, my son," God said, "whom can you tell?" Touché, big guy.

Except for not being a sinner and all, I was like that priest: such an amazing experience that I had to keep secret! When I got back to school, I assumed my place as the quiet kid, and didn't tell anyone that I had just played the lead in a show with all sorts of famous people. I wanted to tell them how cool I was, but I knew I couldn't. If I ever got picked on at school, I wanted to say, "Oh yeah, well I just hung out with Julia Roberts, so suck on that!" But alas, I kept it inside.

It was well worth it, though. Those days at camp shaped me into the person that I am today—not because of the famous people, but because of the experiences. The other kids. The counselors. Getting to be a normal kid for a week was exhilarating. It far outweighed any of the negative stuff that I went through, living with HIV. That's why I say that I wouldn't change my life for the world. Every tough step has made way for 50 amazing experiences, ones that I wouldn't trade for anything.

CHAPTER SEVEN

MY life with HIV continued to be filled with both amazing and difficult experiences. I was getting the hang of keeping that side of my life tucked away and trying to live a normal life as a kid. Still, I had to be very aware of my surroundings in my normal life. For example, when anyone in my school got the chickenpox, I got two weeks off of school so I could get the VZIG shots and be quarantined until all the germs cleared out of school. Doctor's orders. Of course, I had to do all my work from home, but it was pretty sweet to get to do it on my own schedule in my PJs, and hang out with my mom the rest of the day. You know, I always felt sorry for home-schooled kids, but come to think of it, maybe they have it pretty good. All I knew was that I loved those days off. Here, being different was awesome and so was sleeping in. My classmates and some of my teachers wondered why I was out of school for these periods of time, and we would just use the old standby—"she has a heart problem."

While chickenpox did give me random school vacations from time to time, it has also been a source of panic for me throughout my whole life. I never got chickenpox as a kid (knock on wood...no really, do it). Once, when I was a tiny little kid—after I was infected with HIV, but before we knew about it—my sister got chickenpox. My parents actually wanted me to play with her so that I would get it and could be done with it. I played with my speckly sister, and wouldn't you know it, my damaged little immune system came through for me. I never got it. The downside to this is that my body has never had the chance to build antibodies to chickenpox, so I'm particularly susceptible to it as an adult. Hence, my ears perk up and my heartbeat quickens when I hear someone mention chickenpox. If anyone around me gets it, then I have a date with the VZIG shots.

Between the chickenpox vacations and my frequent hospital visits, I'm pretty sure that I had a reputation as a slacker and my parents had a reputation for being irresponsible. If only we could tell people. At that point I lived in genuine fear that my family would be shunned if the community found out. It was a time when stigma thrived, and false information was, well, viral. HIV was seen as a deadly disease, and people still didn't know that you couldn't get it from being around someone who had it. We had heard stories of kids being banned from their schools and families ousted from their communities simply because people were uneducated.

I could never let it slip. I could never even let on that I knew a thing or two about HIV. One day at school I was standing in line on the playground after recess. The kid in front of me moved ahead and I wasn't paying attention, and created a big gap in the line. The girl behind me said, "Come on, move up. He don't got AIDS."

I looked at her, dumbfounded. Speechless, I just stared at her. Did she really think that you could get AIDS by standing next to someone in line? We were only 10 years old, but shouldn't she know better? And why on earth was she so eager to get back to class?!

I wanted to say to her, 'Um, excuse me. I actually couldn't get AIDS from him if he had it, even if I touched him and gave him a hug and a kiss. It's not possible. It's actually only spread through body fluids, through sexual contact, IV drug use, and in rare and very unfortunate cases, through tainted blood products. That last one, that's actually how I got it. But don't worry. We can still be friends because you can't catch it from me. It's an honest mistake, but I'm glad we had this talk. Let's go to the tire swing.'

Alas, I had to keep my mouth shut. If I used that opportunity to educate her on how HIV is actually transmitted, I would have blown my cover. So I just played dumb. Which I hate doing because I always like being right! But I had to maintain this façade of not knowing much about HIV. It would be rather suspicious if I started spouting off facts about HIV; kids weren't supposed to know that stuff.

I got pretty good at playing dumb. When we learned about HIV/AIDS in school, I always had this fear that somehow someone could tell that I knew all about this. So I played dumb. Well, apparently, I played too dumb on one particular day in the school. Our physical education teacher also taught health class, and she happened to know about my status. She was one of the privileged few privy to this knowledge in those early years. She was teaching the class that HIV doesn't stay alive in the air after a certain period of time. Well, I was committed to keeping up my act of "girl who doesn't know anything about HIV," so I raised my hand to ask a very well-rehearsed question.

"Yes, Jamie?"

"Well, if the virus doesn't survive in the air, how come doctors don't just 'air out' people's blood if they have HIV?"

I overshot that one on the scale of dumb questions, because my classmates just laughed at me. So I had successfully maintained my status of "girl who doesn't know anything about HIV," and as a bonus, elevated myself to "girl who asks ridiculously stupid questions." Ehhh, you win some, you lose some.

I learned to calibrate my playing-dumb façade and managed to maintain my anonymity throughout school. While I had this secret second life, I was still living as a relatively normal kid. I got used to telling white lies about having a heart condition. It wasn't until the sixth grade that having HIV became very real for me.

Every sixth grader in my county goes to Outdoor Education camp. It's a rite of passage for elementary school kids. Starting at the beginning of fifth grade, everybody began talking about sixth grade camp. We watched in awe as the upperclassmen (sixth graders) loaded onto the bus for a week of camp. When they came back, we fed on the week's gossip. Who kissed whom? Who got their period for the first time? Who got an allergic reaction to nature? We were mesmerized.

It was a big deal.

When my sixth grade year came along, my class was rapt with anticipation. It was finally our year to go to camp. I joined in the frenzied conversations of what people were packing, what they would wear to the dance, and who wanted to be bunkmates. In the back of my head, though, was a lurking fear. I had managed to keep my HIV status under wraps for this long, but how on earth was I going to pull it off while spending day in and day out with my classmates? They would notice that I took medicine all the time. On top of that, my medication regimen would require the camp nurse to get a crash course in mixing meds. I'm sure that's not what she signed up for. We would have to tell the camp administrators, and who knows how they would react?

All in all, I was petrified. I desperately wanted to join in this rite of passage with my friends, but the risks were too high. If they messed up my meds, I was in trouble. If kids started to ask questions . . . trouble. My parents and I discussed what to do and finally decided that it was best for me to stay behind. While I was devastated to have to sit it out, I was secretly relieved that I wouldn't have to risk being discovered or having my medicines messed up.

On camp day, all my classmates came to school with their luggage all packed up and ready to go. I showed up as I normally did, with my backpack. I watched everyone load onto the bus, in a hyper pre-adolescent frenzy. They were all headed to sixth grade camp, and I was headed to . . . fifth grade.

Yes. Not only did I have to watch longingly as all my friends left me for a week, but I had to face the utter humiliation of being a weird sixth grader stuck in the fifth grade. My teachers assigned me a week's worth of homework to do on various nature topics. I sat in the back of the class, next to the teacher's desk and quietly did my work while she taught. My saving grace was that I was with my favorite elementary school teacher, Mrs. Harner. She let me help her with some of her lessons so I didn't feel like a dweeb. She made me feel like I was the cool older kid in her class, rather than the weirdo girl who couldn't go to camp.

The week went by; it was quiet and pretty lonely, but otherwise tolerable. At the end of the week, my fellow sixth graders were set to return from their nature adventure. I was so excited to see everyone! I had missed them so much and I was so ready for things to get back to normal.

At the end of the day, I went to the cafeteria to wait for the buses. I was most excited to see my best friend, Kerri. I was so used to seeing her every day at school, and most weekend days at each others' houses. After a long week, I had missed her so much. The buses pulled up and I excitedly got up and went to the front door of school. I stood there as everyone filed off the bus, saying hi to my friends as they disembarked. When I saw Kerri, we ran towards each other to say hello and give each other hugs. What came next was unexpected. In addition to my feelings of excitement, I became immediately overwhelmed with . . . I don't even know what. I completely lost it and started bawling as we were hugging. I was thrilled to have my friend back, but also sad and mad that I had to miss what they had just experienced. All my emotions of the week just spilled out right there on the curb. I was a snotty sobbing mess. I didn't realize until that moment how hard it was for me to be so far removed—literally and figuratively—from normal life.

Kerri started crying too, and we ended up making an awful scene. The teachers tucked us away in the school office to let us compose ourselves. We both just wanted to hang out like we always did, so the teacher called my mom to see if I could go home with Kerri's mom. They probably would have done anything to get us to stop crying. My mom of course said yes, and Kerri and I got to hang out and reconnect after a long week.

By the time school came around on Monday I had recovered, and was no longer a blubbering mess. Life was back to normal and I could go back to being a sixth grader.

Years later, I finally got my 6th grade camp experience as a counselor in the 11th grade. By that time, I could handle my meds myself, therefore making it safe for me to be away from home. I counseled my little cabin of girls that week and got the experience I had missed out on years earlier. At which point, I realized that if I wasn't at Hole in the Wall, camping was not fun at all. Yech.

CHAPTER EIGHT

OVER the years, I typically had great success on each medication. I responded well, with minimal side-effects, and my numbers looked relatively good. I switched medications only when my numbers started to dip or when a better medication came out. When I was in middle school, a new medication called 3TC was approved for Phase I clinical drug trials in pediatric patients. It held the promise of results never seen before in young patients. It seemed like a good option for me, and the folks at NIH wanted me to try it out. I began the protocol as I normally did, with a fresh baseline of testing. Thankfully, it didn't involve LPs. I began the 3TC regimen and we waited to see how I would respond.

At school, I began to feel more and more tired. I didn't have the energy to do everything my friends did, and I ended up laying low for a while. It was approaching Christmas, and my mom planned a vacation for her, Heather, and me. We had always wanted to go to Hawaii in the winter to see the humpback whales, and now was the time to do it.

The three of us flew out right after Christmas and began our adventure. We had researched the best whale watching expeditions, and decided on a company that had a tiny little pontoon boat. We piled into the boat with a few other vacationers and set out on the high seas.

"Look for a spout of water," the guide told us. We all scanned the horizon to catch a glimpse of a whale. After about 30 minutes we saw some spouts in the distance, and the guide turned the boat in that direction. We got as close as we could get without scaring them away, and stopped to see what they would do.

A couple of whales crested the water about 100 yards out and flipped their tails out of the water. We all watched, waiting for one to do a breach, jumping out of the water. A few minutes later they gave us quite the show, flipping their tails and jumping into full breaches. We all clapped, cheered, and snapped photos. It was amazing.

Then they quieted down and laid low in the water. We kept watching, waiting to see if one would do an encore performance for us. Just then, we saw a spout of water shoot up about 20 feet from the boat.

"Whoa!" we all yelled, not expecting them to come that close. He dipped back down and came even closer. He crested the water, and we saw the barnacles on his back. Then he came even closer and popped his head up at the edge of the boat. We could have reached out and touched him.

We didn't know if we were supposed to be scared or excited; I went with excited. He swam around the boat and dipped directly underneath, clearly playing with us.

"Here, put on a mask, quick!" the guide yelled.

We all did as instructed and put on diving masks.

"Okay, come over here. Put your head in the water and I'll hold your feet."

What!? You're going to feed us to the whales?

"Okay!" we said, clearly okay with being fed to the whales.

I put on my mask and plunged my face into the water. No more than 10 feet away from me was the most magnificent humpback whale I had ever seen. Okay, really it was the only humpback whale I had ever seen until that day, but it WAS magnificent. I looked right at it, into its huge eyeball. It just hovered there, looking right back at me. It was incredible. I would have stayed down there forever had I not needed to breath and such.

We all took a turn dipping our heads in the water to get a close-up look at the whale. Finally, the whales had had their fun and swam away.

"You guys just got mugged," the guide said. "That was ridiculous. I've never seen them come that close before."

We rode back elated from our whale mugging experience. It was truly the highlight of any vacation to date. For the rest of our time there, we did the normal tourist thing, lying by the pool, shopping, eating at our favorite restaurants. Every day I became exhausted by the afternoon and took a nap in the condo. I was running out of steam more and more easily.

We flew home in time to start school after the winter break. A couple of weeks later, my mom and dad told me that we were going on another trip, this time to the Bahamas—just the three of us. What a bonus! This vacationing was getting great!

We packed our bags and the three of us headed down to the sunny Bahamas. I had my mom and dad all to myself, and it was wonderful. We swam in the luxurious pools all day long, and walked down to the white sand beaches. The water was crystal clear, like nothing I had ever seen before. My dad gave me money to get my hair braided on the beach.

One afternoon we went to a jewelry store in town, a common stop for us in any setting. My mom went into every jewelry store in every place we visited. We looked at the ruby rings, which were a specialty of that particular store.

"Sweetie," my dad said, "I want you to pick out something special."

"What? Really?" I looked at my mom, and she smiled and nodded her head.

"I can pick out anything?"

"Yeah."

"Even one of those ruby rings?"

"Yeah. We want you to have something special from our trip. And you should pick out something too," my dad said to my mom.

I looked through all the rings and decided on one with a row of rubies. My dad bought it and I walked out, proudly wearing it on my finger.

"Thank you guys!" I said, hugging them.

"You're welcome. We love you so much."

After an incredible few days spending quality time together, we headed back home. Back to reality. When I returned to school, one of my classmates asked me where I had been.

"My mom and dad and I went to the Bahamas."

"Geez. You just got back from Hawaii, and then you go to the Bahamas? I want your life," she said.

I just laughed.

The feeling of exhaustion continued, and my numbers were steadily declining. My mom asked the NIH staff what they were going to do.

"Well, we just need to keep her on this medication for another three months to get a complete data set. Then we can think about switching her to another one."

"To hell with that. You're switching her right now. She's fading and you guys know it. Put her on a different medication now."

That was all the persuading it took. I quickly transitioned to another medication and my numbers began to come back up again. Luckily, I bounced back and responded very well. My energy came back, and my numbers looked much better. I felt like myself again.

CHAPTER NINE

"HEY Jamie, do you want to go to this celebrity event in California?" my mom asked me one day.

"Ummmm, yeah? What is it?"

"It's the Pediatric AIDS Foundation. They invited us to go to their annual picnic this year."

"That's awesome! When do we go?"

"In June. And they want you to sing."

"What? Why do they want me to sing?"

"Because the people from NIH told them that you are an amazing singer, and they want you to perform."

"Wow, okay. What am I supposed to sing?"

"You need to think of a song to sing and Richard Marx's band will be playing back-up for you."

Well how about that.

The Pediatric AIDS Foundation was started by Elizabeth Glaser in 1988 in an effort to save her children. Elizabeth was infected with HIV from a blood transfusion while giving birth to her daughter, Ariel. Elizabeth unknowingly passed the virus on to her children, Ariel and Jake. When Ariel died at the young age of seven, Elizabeth banded together with her two best friends, Susie Zeegen and Susan DeLaurentis, to form what is now called the Elizabeth Glaser Pediatric AIDS Foundation (EGPAF). Elizabeth and her friends set out to give hope to children facing HIV by advocating for lifesaving research and treatment. She fought tirelessly to bring the issue to the table and fund HIV drug treatment for children. Elizabeth lost her own battle with HIV in 1994, but her vision lives on in the work the foundation does today, all over the world.

I was lucky enough to join the EGPAF family as a young teenager, with that invitation to join them for their annual picnic. When we arrived in Los Angeles, the EGPAF staff met us to review the itinerary for the weekend.

"This afternoon we're bringing you to the venue to do a sound check with Richard and the band. Then tomorrow, we'll bring you to the event early so you can do some press interviews to talk about your experiences. Then, at the end of the event, we'll gather you and the other kids on stage to say some remarks. Sound good?"

Um sure, just one question—whose life am I living right now?

"Yes," I said, "sounds good."

"And you don't have to give your full name when you talk to the press. Or you can make up a name. Up to you."

"Okay."

We later drove over to the venue to meet Richard and the band and do a run-through of the song I was singing, *I Can See Clearly Now*. The sound guys were setting up and we all went backstage to wait.

"This is my wife Cynthia," Richard said, introducing me to Cynthia Rhodes.

"Nice to meet you," I said. First, I'm singing with a famous band, and now I'm hanging out with Penny from Dirty Dancing? This just keeps getting better and better!

After a few successful run-throughs of the song, we headed back to the hotel. The next morning, I was a nervous wreck. Stage fright was steadily kicking in. We headed over to the event with the other families and when we arrived, the event was in full swing and the grounds were packed with people. All these people had shown up to support kids like me. All these people were on my side. It was an amazing feeling.

I ran around the event, meeting celebrities, getting pictures taken, and being utterly star struck. My mom and I were waiting in line to get an iced coffee when we heard a deep sultry voice behind us say, "Hello, ladies." We turned around to see Jack Nicholson waiting in line behind us.

"Hi," we said back, trying to keep our composure. No big deal.

The amazing thing was that they all thought I was the cool one. Um seriously, Tom Hanks. You're Forrest Gump and you're telling me how great I am?

The support and compassion they showed was overwhelming. These people had taken time out of their schedules to show up and support the efforts of saving our lives. Incredible.

The event was a blast, but I was a nervous wreck about having to sing my song in front of all these important people. Performance time was coming up and I was a ball of nerves. I went backstage and joined the band as we got ready to go on.

"Don't worry," Richard said, "you'll do great."

Okay, famous recording artist. Easy for you to say.

We got up on stage and I went on autopilot. I couldn't look at the crowd. Instead, I stared at the mountain in the background the entire time. When it was over, I scurried offstage to finally breathe a sigh of relief, still my favorite feeling.

At the end of the event, I went back on stage to join the group for closing remarks. Flanked by my peers, other kids with HIV, I listened to the amazing words of hope that everyone shared. Paul Glaser spoke of his wife's courageous disclosure in a time when AIDS was still very much stigmatized, and her incredible dedication to her mission. Ted Danson and Mary Steenburgen, strong supporters of EGPAF, spoke about the amazing work the foundation had done. They talked about cures and finding new medicines for us. The message of hope was loud and clear and I got up feeling optimistic as ever.

When the event came to a close, Ted and Mary walked over to me.

"Your story is amazing, Jamie," Mary said. "And

you have a beautiful voice."

"Thank you. That's so nice!"

"You really did great," Ted said. "It's amazing to see how healthy you are, after what you've been through."

"Thanks. You guys are amazing too. What you do for the foundation is really cool. It really means a lot."

We went on to chat about the basics, where we lived, our families.

"Hey, I just got one of those electric cars," Ted said.

"What? I didn't even know they made electric cars," I replied.

"Yeah, it's pretty cool. You want to drive it?"

"Um . . . I don't have my driver's license."

"That's okay. We'll just take it up through the hills."

"Um, yeah. Let me go ask my parents."

I ran over to find my parents in the crowd. "Hey Mom and Dad, can I go drive Ted Danson's electric car?"

"What?"

"Yeah, he just asked if I wanted to drive his new car. Can I?"

"Um, okay. When?"

"Right now."

"Uhhhhh. Okay. Be careful!"

I ran back over to them. "Okay, yeah I can go. My parents said yes."

"Great! You ready?"

With that, Ted and I walked out of the event to his car. He drove it out of the parking lot, away from the event traffic, and pulled over to switch sides with me.

I got in the driver's side and checked everything out. Please don't crash Ted Danson's car. Please don't crash Ted Danson's car, I repeated in my head. I pulled onto the road and started to drive up the hills of Brentwood.

"You can go faster," he said.

"Okay," I said, nervously. I pressed on the gas a little more.

"Go faster. You gotta see what this thing does. When we crest this hill up here, floor it."

"Okay . . ." I had no idea what I was doing. As instructed, I floored it when we got to the top of the hill, and it took off like a rocket.

"Whoa!" I said. "This is awesome!"

"Yeah, I told you!" he said.

I sped around for a few more miles and then turned back to rejoin Mary and my family.

"Thank you so much. For everything," I said to both of them. We exchanged information, hugged goodbye, and went on our way.

The weekend wound down and we headed home to Pennsylvania to transition back into our non-HIV lives. What an amazing experience that I couldn't tell anyone about!

A few weeks later, I got a package in the mail from Ted and Mary. It was a beautiful necklace and a note saying how great it was to meet each other. I wore my necklace as a secret reminder of the amazing experience I'd just had. More importantly, it reminded me of the incredible people who were out there, fighting for our lives. People who took a break from the limelight and gave to others. People like Ted and Mary and Elizabeth, who cared enough to do something.

CHAPTER TEN

ONE of the keys to ensuring that HIV therapies are effective is sticking to the very strict dosage and timing protocol. Back in the early days, this was not a pop-a-pill-a-day disease. Some drugs had to be taken every eight hours on the dot. Some had to be taken with food, some on an empty stomach. Some were in pill form, some were injections, and some were liquid. Some had to be mixed right before taking. Some could only be taken facing West at dusk when the moon was in the seventh house. Well, almost. These medications required a great deal of discipline and precision to ensure that they were effective.

One of my first drug protocols should have earned my mom an honorary chemistry degree. This one, DDI, required an arsenal of supplies for mixing. We would come home from NIH with bags of supplies; truly, we could be running a drug cartel out of our backyard. I sat down at our kitchen bar, and watched my mom as she prepped her workspace, making sure everything was clean. She pulled out the vial of liquid, a vial of powder, and syringes. It's a good thing we lived in the woods at this point, because anyone passing by our window would have thought she was teaching me the family business of being a drug lord.

My mom drew up the liquid into the syringe and tapped it until she got every last tiny little bubble to the top. This was no quick tap tap—these bubbles clung to the sides of the syringe for dear life. The trick was to apply enough force to get them to float up without creating new bubbles. When all the bubbles were tapped out, she pushed the plunger up to get the air out of the top. She then stuck that syringe into a vial of powder, mixing the two. Next it was shake and bake time, minus the bake. The goal here was to get all the powder dissolved into the liquid. My mom alternated between shaking and rolling the vial in her hands. The whole process took about 30 minutes and it had to be perfect.

My mom instilled a healthy love of—no, an obsession with—jewelry in me at a young age. She wore her rings and bracelets all day, including when she mixed my meds. As she shook the vial, her bracelets clanked together. It also clattered against her rings when she rolled it in her hands. Those were the sounds of a mother's pure dedication to her child.

DDI was to be taken every eight hours on an empty stomach. I also had to take two tablespoons of Maalox before each dose. The kitchen timer was our most useful tool during these years. I took the chalky Maalox exactly two minutes before taking the DDI. Maalox. Timer. DDI (bitter clear liquid in two teaspoons of apple juice). Timer set for 30 minutes. When the timer buzzed, I could eat. I would watch the timer with my snack in front of me, desperately wanting the minutes to tick by faster. I was, and still am, a professional snacker, so those fasting times were no fun for me.

On another drug protocol, I had to take a dose in the middle of the night. My mom got everything ready and brought me my meds at three in the morning. Most of the time, I wouldn't even wake up; I had many a delirious conversation with my mom during this drug protocol.

Then there were the IL-2 years. Our bodies actually make IL-2, or Interleukin-2, to produce cells that fight off infections. It basically helps our immune system work well. It was thought that HIV positive people would benefit from receiving high doses of IL-2. Why not? The staff at NIH were very excited about this new protocol, partly because it was only given for a one-week span every other month. The downside was that it had to be injected twice a day for that week, and it had wicked side effects. It created an immune response in the body, basically mimicking the flu.

Patients had to be very healthy to start this protocol, so I was a prime candidate. There was only one other patient on this protocol, and I signed up to be number two. I was terrified to have to give myself shots, but this treatment was so promising it was hard to pass up.

It meant the possibility that I wouldn't have to take pills every day for the rest of my life. At this point, I was a senior in high school and the thought of getting a break from taking meds every day was a welcome idea.

In preparation for this protocol, I made a visit to NIH so they could gather some preliminary lab work. My mom and I checked in for the day as usual, and went back with the nurse for labs. I had to get blood drawn several times throughout the day, so they decided to place an IV. While I was a pro at blood draws, I absolutely hated IVs. It was not uncommon for me to get so worked up that I passed out cold, thanks to my residual heart issues, low pressure, and nerves. Still, I was getting better at it and had learned to look away and not focus on the IV.

I sat down in the treatment room chair and the nurse—a new nurse whom I had never met—got all her supplies ready. My mom sat down next to me and promptly began talking to me about what we were going to look for at the mall when we were done. I started to answer her but didn't take my eyes off the nurse, who was still on the other side of the room.

Mom tapped my arm. "Hey," she said, "look at me. Don't worry about that. Do you want to see if Nordstrom is having one of their shoe sales today?"

This woman knew how to get my attention.

"Yes!" I lit up at that thought.

"Good. Me too. Where do you want to eat dinner tonight?"

"I don't know. We could go to—"

"Okay, Jamie are you ready?" the nurse said as she

walked over with all her supplies.

"Yeah." I looked at my mom.

"You'll do fine," my mom said. "Just look at me and take deep breaths."

The nurse looked at the top of my hand for a good vein.

"Can you look on my arm first? I really don't like having IVs in my hand."

It was true. I absolutely hated having IVs in my hand.

"You have good veins in your hand, but I can look in your arm."

I was relieved, thinking that she would look in the crook of my elbow, where I always had labs drawn. Instead, she looked at the side of my wrist, about five inches down from my thumb. I had never had an IV placed there before and I was not excited about this new plan. The nurse found a huge vein and decided she would try that one.

I didn't argue because I had already bugged her about not using my hand, but I was not looking forward to this.

She put on her gloves and tied the tourniquet around my arm. She cleaned my wrist with alcohol. I was squeezing my mom's hand already.

"Okay, ready?'

No.

"One."

No, I don't like this.

"Two."

Yeah, this is a bad idea.

"Three."

I squeezed my mom's hand so hard as she stuck the needle in. It felt like the needle filled my entire wrist. I was trying to take deep breaths to calm myself down, but the pain kept getting worse. I kept getting more and more upset and unnerved.

"Jamie, calm down," they were telling me.

I started to hear them as if I were in a tunnel.

"Jamie. Look at me."

They were getting louder.

"Jamie. Stay with us."

I was fading.

"Jamie!"

"Sweetie, open your eyes!"

"Come on, Jamie!"

"She's seizing. We need help in here!"

Darkness.

When I woke up I was in a bed with an oxygen mask on my face, heart monitors stuck to my chest, and a blood pressure cuff on my arm.

"There she is."

"How are you feeling?"

My mom was holding my hand. She leaned over and hugged me. I was exhausted. Drained of all my energy, I just lay there, scared by what had just happened.

A crowd of nurses and doctors were around the bed, making sure I was okay.

"Okay, let's try it again," the young nurse said.

"No, she needs a break." This time it wasn't my mom piping in. It was a nurse I'd never met named

Shannon. Shannon knew her stuff and she knew that I needed a break.

"Give her a rest and we'll try again later."

I was so relieved that I could just rest and recover. I stayed snuggled in that bed for the rest of the day. People came in to check on me periodically. Later, Shannon came back and got my IV in with no trouble. I looked at her and thought, *I like this one.*

This protocol required that I be admitted to the hospital for the duration of the week because they needed to closely monitor my reaction to the new medicine. My mom and I packed our bags and set out for the long stay at NIH. We made up a story for school about being out because of my heart.

We arrived at NIH and checked in. After we got settled, the first thing I had to do was get an IV. I was not too excited for this, given my last experience, but I felt much better when I saw Shannon come into my room. She was my nurse for the day, and I was so relieved. She knew my history with IVs and I knew she would take care of me.

"How about we try something different?" she suggested.

"Like not getting an IV?"

"Not quite what I was thinking. Do you have headphones or something to distract you? You could listen to music while we do it and then you won't have to focus on the IV."

"That's a great idea," my mom said. "I have your headphones in the car, and you just got that Seal CD."

I was slightly obsessed with Kiss From a Rose at this

time.

My mom ran down to get my headphones and we tried it out. It took a couple of times to get the IV in successfully, but it was so much easier for me with something else to focus on. And a major bonus: I didn't pass out or have a seizure. Shannon was a genius!

"You did great!" she said. "Was it better this time?"

"Yes, a lot better."

I looked down at the IV in my arm and inspected it closely. I was careful not to move my arm much because I was afraid of ruining it. Shannon watched me as I gingerly looked at it.

"You know, there isn't a needle in there anymore," she said.

"There's not?"

"No. The needle comes out. There's only a little plastic tube in there now. You can even bend your arm a little bit."

"Oh. That makes me feel so much better! I was afraid I was going to poke a hole through my vein if I bent my arm."

She smiled.

"Yeah, most people think the needle stays in, but it doesn't."

When Shannon told me that, my anxiety practically went away. I felt so much better, knowing that I didn't have a needle stuck in my arm.

Starting that day, I got two IL-2 shots each day. After the first one, all we had to do was wait. Wait to see if I got those nasty flu-like side effects, and wait to see if the drug would be effective against the HIV. Just a few hours into it, we got the answer to the first question. The flu-like side effects came on like a flood. Within 24 hours I was confined to the bed, feeling like I had been hit by a truck. I had a fever, the chills, and my whole body ached. I was miserable. But at the same time, I was very hopeful. I thought that if I was having such severe side effects, that must mean that the drug was working, right? It would take few more months to determine if that was the case, but I got through it, hopeful that it was.

CHAPTER ELEVEN

I was growing up and getting fairly good at balancing my two lives. Camp filled my HIV life with joy and even a sense of normalcy. And I got pretty good at transitioning smoothly back to normal life. Still, I wondered what it would be like to merge the two. How would it feel to just tell someone that I was HIV positive? How would they react? What would it be like not to have to keep this secret? Apart from talking to people in the medical world and at camp, I had yet to know the answers to these questions.

It was time for me to find out. I was tired of lying. I knew that I shouldn't feel ashamed of being HIV positive, but how else could I feel when I had to keep it a secret? I struggled with this balance of keeping the secret to protect myself, and not feeling shame because of it. No one should have to feel shame about being HIV positive, but the reality was—and continues to be—that the shame and fear exist. Still, I was getting fed up with keeping secrets.

On one of our many trips to England, my family visited a magnificent cathedral. This was one of our favorite things to do; ironic, because we were never a church-going family. We were only religious in the tourism sense when we visited churches in England. If our churches here were that beautiful and had gift shops, things might have been different. In all seriousness, our spirituality growing up didn't fit in a traditional religious setting, so visiting these cathedrals in England was that much more exciting.

During one such visit, my mom asked if I wanted the priest to pray for me. I had just experienced a dip in my CD4 counts, and I think my mom felt like we needed all the reinforcement we could get. I said sure, why not? I'm always up for new things. But this would mean that we would sort of have to tell this priest that I was HIV positive, right? Well, that's new.

We approached the priest and my mom said, "My daughter is HIV positive and it would mean a lot if you could say a prayer for her." He looked at me and said, "Of course." He took our hands and said a prayer, asking God to keep me healthy. As he was praying, I was sort of looking around thinking *Is this really happening? I'm not really sure what to do here. Do I curtsy? Shake his hand?* The novelty of telling a perfect stranger that I was HIV positive and praying with a priest were both pretty much uncharted territory for me. Big day: two new things. It was truly a leap of faith.

Afterwards, I felt relieved that he didn't react

negatively, and even better, he was very compassionate towards me. It was a great test case, because had things gone wrong, I would have the whole Atlantic Ocean to protect me from him (or to protect him from my mom). Thankfully though, it was a great experience and I came home hopeful that maybe I would eventually be able to tell anyone. Even if they were American and not of-the-cloth.

Back stateside, I was in my senior year of high school. I had made great friends and I wanted to test the waters to see how people would react to my real life. We were nearing the end of the year and I just wanted my friends to know who I really was before we all went our separate ways. I also thought that my classmates should know what was out there as we moved on, went to college, and started our lives. No one would have guessed in a million years that I was HIV positive. I stayed relatively healthy and didn't have to take too much time off of school.

I wanted people to know that they didn't have to be afraid of people with HIV. At the same time, I wanted people to know that it was out there and they had to protect themselves. So I decided that I wanted to tell my whole senior class. Looking back, the mere thought of that terrifies me, but I was committed to doing this. People needed to know that HIV didn't just happen to "other" people. That being from a small town does not make you immune to the realities of life. And I needed to free myself from this secret life.

It was time to test the waters and see what it was like to tell people. Coincidentally, as if the universe knew what I was planning, I got a phone call from the Oprah Winfrey Show asking if I wanted to be on the show about people living with HIV. They had gotten my name from the hospital, and thought I would be a good addition to their program. I agreed. If I was going to do this, I might as well do it in style. Go big or go home.

The producer called to get all the details of my story up to that point. She was excited to hear how well I was doing, because they wanted to make it a show focused on hope. That worked; I like hope, and that's exactly the message I wanted to convey.

Since more than a couple of people watch Oprah, I knew there was no turning back. It would get out. No more secrets, no more, 'I have a heart defect.' This was it. Thus, my decision to do the show was naturally accompanied by my decision to go public to my high school class.

I traveled to Chicago, ready for my big debut. I was going to tape the show, which would be aired after I addressed my high school. This was good. I was doing the right thing. People needed to know this stuff—at least that's what I kept telling myself. I couldn't turn back now, I had already ordered room service in the complimentary hotel suite.

On the morning of the show, a car brought my mom and me to the studio, and I did the whole hair and make-up thing. Had I known this was so official, I would have demanded some white lilies and green M&M's. I should have milked this thing for all it was worth. Hindsight . . .

I was a ball of nerves and excitement. I had never done anything like this before, but I had to do it. I wanted to tell people my story. The fact that someone as famous as Oprah also wanted to get this message out was so encouraging.

We were on the set with a few other people with HIV who were there to tell their stories as well. I had yet to meet Ms. Winfrey, but I was sure that she had read my bio and knew what a fabulous story I had to tell. When she entered the studio, the audience went crazy. Some people cried. No really—that actually happens. It was all very exciting.

She welcomed the audience and started speaking with everyone before taping began. Fun fact of the day: the audience members don't know the topic or the guest when they line up for tickets. Oprah told them that today, we were going to talk about HIV and hear from some survivors.

After looking under their chairs and not finding car keys, the audience members came up bewildered, asking in disbelief, 'You mean I don't get a new Ford Edge?' 'We aren't meeting a celebrity? And we have to hear about AIDS? What an F---ing drag!'

This point was not lost on Ms. Winfrey, either, who jokingly said, "I know, you were hoping for Tom Cruise! Sorry!"

Um, seriously? Have we met? Because I'm kind of a big deal, according to your complimentary fruit basket in the hotel room.

Off to a swimmingly good start, we began filming the actual show. I was excited to tell my story of hope.

Oprah started off by interviewing two adults who had acquired HIV as adults through unprotected sex and IV drug use. The first man devoted his life to exercising and running marathons after he found out his status. It was a great story of perseverance and determination. A few minutes later, she moved on to her next guest, a woman whose life was turned upside down after she found out. She told the audience about being incapacitated and not being able to use the bathroom on her own. My heart went out to her, but I was also thinking, *Um, that's not very hopeful*. It's actually kind of depressing. That's not what we were all there to talk about. We were supposed to give our message of optimism and strength.

That's fine, I thought. *We'll spend a few moments hearing this sad story, and then we'll move on to more uplifting stories*. A few moments turned into what seemed like the majority of the show. Oprah continued to ask questions about the woman feeling sick and depressed. There wasn't even a hopeful end to her story, it was just sad. Why were we spending all this time talking about depressing things when this was supposed to be a hopeful show? It certainly wasn't helping my outlook on life at that very moment.

It was finally time to hear my story. Whew, I thought, I'll turn this thing around. Oprah introduced my story and they showed a few pictures of me as a young kid up on the screen. Everyone "awwwwwwwed" at how cute I was, naturally. After the introduction, Oprah turned to me and said, "So Jamie, what was it like to tell your classmates that you were HIV positive?"

Ummmmmmmmm . . . I was in a bit of a pickle here, so I answered as best as I could and said, "Well, I haven't told them yet, but by the time this airs, I will have made a speech to my graduating class." She asked me a couple of basic questions, and then moved on to someone else. *Wait, that's it?* I thought. *Don't you want to hear about how healthy I am? I beat the odds! I get kittens and stuff!* Nope. I was done. I guess I wasn't that interesting.

I went away thinking, Well, Chicago is pretty, but I'm not really sure what the point of all that was. I would have liked the chance to say more about how lucky I was. and how everyone should get tested. What I thought was going to be a show about hope turned into an exploitation of someone else's darkest hours. It wasn't the message that I had signed up to tell. At least I got a free mug out of it. And that fruit basket was lovely.

Back in Gettysburg, it was time to start planning my big announcement. I knew that if I was going to do this, I would need some reinforcement. I needed to tell some of my close friends to get some allies on my side. This would also serve as a trial run for the real deal; if my good friends didn't take it well, then the deal was off. I started slowly. I spent a lot of time with two of my best friends, Miranda and Joel. They were dating, and the three of us were like the Three Musketeers. Although, looking back, maybe I was just the third wheel? Oh man. Sorry guys. No really, we were great friends and I wanted to tell them the whoel story about myself.

I started with Miranda. We sat on my couch one afternoon after school.

"So I kind of want to tell you something."

"Okay. You can tell me anything."

I started from the beginning and told her about my heart defect, my surgery, and finding out that I was HIV positive. Miranda was always a quiet and gentle person, and she just listened. She quietly said "Oh my God," or "Wow" throughout my story.

"I never would have known," she said.

"I know. I've been really lucky. I've stayed pretty healthy. You're the first person outside of my hospital and camp that I've ever told."

"Wow. I'm honored," she said.

She couldn't have been a better friend. She asked a couple of questions, and most importantly, she gave me a hug. We both cried a little bit. I was so relieved. This was the first time I had ever done this, and it went so well. For the first time in my life, I didn't have to be secretive with someone in my non-HIV life. A weight was lifted off my shoulders, and I was thrilled. It was literally exhilarating. What should I do next? Tell more people!

I wanted to tell Joel next. With Miranda in my corner, I had back-up this time. The three of us got together one day and we told Joel that there was something I wanted him to know about me. He could have been thinking anything at this point; his girlfriend and one of his best girl-friends had something to tell him? This could have gone in so many directions; who knows what was going through his head.

After thoroughly squashing any teenage male fantasy he may have had, I told him the real story. I was still nervous, this only being the second time I'd done this.

"I would have never known," he said. "I can't believe it. It's so great that you're so healthy."

I received the same loving support—hugs, tears, and more encouragement that I might not have to live my life as a secret.

I was two for two and there was no stopping me now. Next up: my friend Joe, who I had just recently started being all romantic with. He was my prom date and I liked him a whole lot. I was upping the ante with this one. I wanted him to know before I told the whole class. I wanted the chance to tell him very clearly that I had never put him in any danger by kissing or hugging him. He is one of the smartest people I know, but I had no idea what he knew—or didn't know—about HIV.

This time we were at Joel's house. Joel and Miranda were there with me; my posse was getting bigger. Joe came over and we sat down in Joel's living room and started what had become known as "The Talk." I told Joe my story from start to finish, emphasizing the fact that he was not at risk of being exposed to the virus by kissing me. I could tell that he was shocked, and that he didn't quite know what to do with this news. It was certainly the last thing he was expecting me to tell him, I'm sure. Having Miranda and Joel there, however, helped bring him back to reality, and reassured him that everything was okay. I was so thankful to have them there; not only did I need their support, but Joe did too.

"I never would have known," he said.

I get that a lot, I thought.

After lots of questions, we were able to put that conversation behind us and move on. Now I had three people in my corner and I was feeling optimistic. Each conversation took a little weight off my shoulders.

It was now time for the real deal—do or die time. I still needed to address my whole class, so my parents and I met with the school superintendent, Dr. Mowery. We gave him our proposal of what I wanted to do. We lived in a small town, and people liked their small town lives. I didn't know how he would feel about this.

His response couldn't have been more wonderful. He was touched to hear my story and incredibly supportive of my wanting to go public. From that point on, we worked together on a plan. Following graduation rehearsal, my senior class would be called in for an assembly, where I would address them and tell my story. Immediately following, I would address all the school's teachers. Yikes.

I wrote a speech and went over it with my parents and Dr. Mowery. We tweaked it here and there and came up with the right combination of my story, facts about HIV, and my advice for my classmates. It was, in a nutshell, "here's my life story and don't be stupid."

Senior year was coming to a close and graduation was drawing near. In addition to the excitement of graduating, I had the growing anxiety of my big announcement. That day of graduation rehearsal, I was a nervous wreck. It was a hot June day, and the school leaders were just trying to get us through one rehearsal—no small feat with 300 seniors who are all wound up. It was like trying to get bumblebees to fly in a straight line. Amidst the chaos, I was a disaster inside. I was feeling more anxiety than I had ever felt before and we were beyond the point of no return. I went through the motions of graduation rehearsal in an anxious daze. I considered making a break for it, but realized that I wouldn't make it very far without passing out (thanks, stupid heart.)

After rehearsal, we had a break for lunch before the assembly time. I went to Hardees with a group of friends, and my anxiety just kept building. Minute by minute, I became more and more of a basket case. Why did I decide to do this anyway? I was graduating, for God's sake! I had successfully kept myself a secret for this long, and I could just go away unnoticed. But now I wanted to tell everybody, and make graduation a big stress ball of angst!? At this point, I just needed to get it over with . . . and run for the hills, if I had to. My timing was no coincidence. If people freaked out and the townsfolk started coming at me with pitchforks, I could just get out of Dodge. Seriously.

Lunch was over, and it was time to report back to school. People were asking each other at lunch why we were having an assembly. No one knew what was coming, and I just played dumb.

When got back to school, everyone started to file in to the auditorium, and I snuck backstage without anyone noticing. Joel, Miranda, and Joe were back there with me. I was so grateful to have them there to help me avoid a breakdown. My parents were there, hidden in the back of the auditorium, where none of the students could see them.

The auditorium was rumbling with chatter as people filed in and took their seats. My short-term goal at this point was to not pass out or throw up. Dr. Mowery took the stage and called for the class's attention.

Oh God.

This was it.

I took the podium, gripping it as if my life depended on it, and started to read my speech.

> Hello. As Dr. Mowery said, I have had a pretty interesting life. As a matter of fact, I've kind of led a double life. Please listen carefully to my story and hopefully you'll learn something. When I was three years old, I had open heart surgery and I received a blood transfusion. That transfusion contained the AIDS virus. When I was ten, I found out that I was HIV positive. What I've learned since then will hopefully help each of you as you go forward in life. I started treatment at the National Institutes of Health, when I was ten, where I have been followed ever since. For almost eight years now, I have taken various medications to keep me well. Right now, I'm on AZT and DDI, as well as IL-2, an experimental drug.

> First, I want to get some basic facts out of the way. AIDS is spread through blood, semen, vaginal secretions, and breast milk. It's never been spread through saliva. You cannot get it by casual contact,

which includes sharing a glass, kissing, holding hands, or using the same bathroom as an HIV-infected person. You CAN get it through any kind of unprotected sex and IV drug use.

Up until now, I've led a secret life. When we found out, my parents were told that I had two years to live, and they decided not to tell anyone except my family so that I could have a fairly normal life, for however long that might be. But surprise! I'm still here.

At this point in my speech, people applauded. It was the first sign I had that people were taking it well. I remember feeling a huge sense of relief as I continued on with my speech.

As I grew up, I decided to stay private about it because I was scared. I was scared of how I would be treated if everyone knew. I was scared that I would be shunned and I wouldn't have any friends. I was scared that people wouldn't listen to the information about AIDS and HIV.

But today, I'm more afraid for all of you. And I'm telling you this now to open your eyes. We think we live in a safe zone where nothing will happen to us, but it's not true. I'm here to say that it can happen to you, if you're not careful. Until now, many of you thought that AIDS and HIV didn't even exist in Gettysburg, that it couldn't affect you, and that you were safe. You have to understand that you are not immune to this. Of the few people I've told in the last few months, one of their main reactions is "I had no idea." No one can tell if the people around them have AIDS just by looking at them.

As you go out into the world, please remember that AIDS doesn't just happen to bad people. You can't look at someone and decide they're safe. You can't think that because someone has a fancy car or dresses well, they can't have AIDS. AIDS does not discriminate—it can happen to anyone, no matter who you are.

From my life of dealing with this, I can offer you one piece of advice. Don't be stupid. Don't use IV drugs, or any other kind for that matter. And, as we've been told a hundred times, abstinence is the only 100% form of protection when it comes to sex. If you decide to have sex, use a condom every time. Another thing that people don't often think about is the use of alcohol regarding AIDS. If you're at a party and you get drunk, you are not going to make sensible decisions and you could end up sleeping with someone you wouldn't have, otherwise. Think about it. When you make the decision to sleep with someone, you may think they're safe, but there is no way to be sure. Just remember this: when you have sex with someone, you are exposing yourself to every other person they have been with. So your one decision has exposed you to more people than you think, and you're taking a huge risk. Your partner might not even know if they have AIDS or not, and if they don't know, there's no way for you to be sure. Bottom line: be smart, be safe, use condoms, and if you think you're at risk, get tested.

There are places you can go for information or to get tested and they even sell home testing kits now. Another thing—get the facts about AIDS if you're unsure of anything because at our age, we all need to know what's going on.

I couldn't help getting this. The course of my life was set for me when I was three. But you guys have a choice, and let me tell you, it's not worth taking the risk. Just remember that the decisions you'll face in the next years will change your life; make sure they're the right ones. As we graduate and go our separate ways, please remember this day. Thank you.

Finishing that speech was like jumping off a bridge without knowing if there was a safety net. How on earth were they going to react to this? They applauded once during my speech, but would they turn against me? Would they not want me at graduation? How would they treat me? Would they do anything to me or my family? I had absolutely no idea.

At my closing remarks, I took a step back from the podium and waited. What happened next was as shocking as it was exhilarating. Applause. Cheering. Standing. I couldn't believe it. I stood there and a huge wave of relief hit me. I had done it, and it had actually gone well. And it wasn't over yet.

One by one, all my classmates came up to the stage to give me a hug. Many of them said thank you. Some of my closest friends met me with tears and huge hugs. I was overwhelmed. I never actually expected people to be sad for me, or this supportive. I stood on stage for what seemed like hours, greeting my classmates one by one. I had never felt this type of support in my life. I realized then that I had underestimated people. The Gettysburg High School Class of '97 surpassed my expectations, and I love and appreciate each and every one of them for that. Social boundaries were obliterated at that moment, and I connected with people I never would have connected with, otherwise. It was one of the best feelings of my life.

If anyone reacted negatively to my announcement, I never knew it. I felt immense relief, but I had one more speech ahead of me, to the teachers. I was so emotionally drained at that point I was truly dreading having to do it all over again to another group. But there really was no turning back now, so I had to do it.

I moved to another room to address the teachers, and this time I had even more back-up. A big group of my friends came with me and sat on stage with me as the teachers filed into the room. It was amazing feeling. Never before had I been with my peers, with them knowing this huge part of my life. I was raw and vulnerable, and amazingly, I was okay.

I could tell that the teachers were very suspicious about why they were being addressed, and by a student, no less. Anyone who is a teacher, or who knows a teacher, knows that they are just as burned-out as students are by the end of the year. Gathering for a mystery meeting was probably the last thing they wanted to do at that point.

I sort of winged this speech. I was so focused on my speech to my classmates that I didn't focus too much on how I would address my teachers. I certainly wasn't there to tell them not to get drunk at a party and sleep with everybody. They should know that by now.

I told my story and focused on getting them to realize that our little town wasn't immune to AIDS. I told them not to judge students, because they never knew what their lives were really like. I also wanted them to know that all their students were living in a world where HIV could happen to them if they weren't careful.

I wrapped up my speech and a very interesting thing happened. Only one or two teachers came up to talk to me. The rest filed out, barely making eye contact. Having just gotten such a warm reception from my classmates, I was pretty surprised not to get the same from my teachers. I can't speculate on why that happened; everyone reacts differently, I was learning. Those who did come up and show their support meant the world to me.

The next day was graduation and I could finally relax and embrace the excitement of this event. It was another sunny day, and the day that every high school kid waited for was finally here. We filed onto the football field in our maroon and white robes, before our families and friends. One row at a time, we got our diplomas and had our proud moment on the stage. When they called my row, I got nervous again—but this time, I was an excited nervous, versus the panicked nervous of the day before. They called my name and I started to walk. As I walked, I looked to my right, and saw that my entire class was standing and cheering for me. I could not believe it. I had no idea that they were going to do this, and it overwhelmed me yet again with a feeling of love and support.

The rest of the day was a blur. Here I was, graduating from high school. A mere ten years ago, we didn't think that I would live to see this day. And to top it all off, I could—for the first time in my life—be honest about who I was. This was the beginning of big things for me. My days of being a high school student, a "kept" person, were over. More importantly, the days of living a secret life were over. For the first time, my HIV- and non-HIV lives were one and the same, and so far, it was amazing.

CHAPTER TWELVE

IN the grand tradition of the American high school senior, my friends and I embarked on our first trip alone: Senior Week. Miranda, Joel, Joe and I packed the car and set out to the exotic and luxurious . . . New Jersey. Not even the maniacal, fist-pumping Jersey of the Jersey shore; we were headed to Cape May. Don't get me wrong, Cape May is a beautiful little town full of Victorian mansions and early bird specials. Perfect for the 50-something-plus crowd. And four high school graduates, apparently. Maybe we were being rebellious in our own intellectual way. Keg stands? Wet T-shirt contests? Forget that. We were going to go on a CATAMARAN! And enjoy a good NOVEL! Crazytown! After a week of good clean elderly fun, we headed back home.

When I got home, my parents and Heather were there to greet me. After I unpacked and settled back in, my mom came to talk to me.

"Hey Sweetie, can you come downstairs for a minute? We need to talk to you."

Oh God. This couldn't be good. My experience with these conversations in the past was that they are kind of a bummer. What the hell else is wrong with me now? Or maybe this was the talk before college about not putting your drink down anywhere?

We walked out to our back porch and sat down with my dad and Heather. Uh oh. What did Heather do? Is she in big trouble?

"Honey, there is something we need to tell you. You know your dad and I have been arguing a lot lately."

It was true. They had argued off and on for a while, but I assumed this was normal for married couples. They rarely argued in front of us, and everything seemed fine for the most part.

"Your dad and I have been working on some of our issues, and have done a lot of talking. We've decided that it would be best to do a trial separation."

"What? Why?" I asked. "Are you guys getting a divorce?"

"Right now we are just separating, and we're going to see how it goes. Your dad is not going to be here during the week, but he'll come back on weekends."

"When is this going to start?" I asked.

"We started it this past week."

"While I was away?"

"Yes."

"But I called every night and no one said anything. What if I had asked to talk to Dad?"

"Well, we would have figured that out if you had

asked."

Man, were they lucky that I was oblivious to minor details, like my dad not living in our house.

"Dad, where are you going to stay during the week?"

"I'll stay at my shop in Maryland."

There was nothing I could say or do. All I could do was cry.

"We never wanted to hurt you girls. This is the best thing for us."

I never thought this would happen to our family. My parents fought, but they always assured us that everything was going to be okay. Until then, our deep dark secret was me, and I naively thought that because my family dealt with health issues, everything else in our lives would remain stable. I was in the spotlight so much that I was blinded to what was really happening around me.

That Sunday evening, I said goodnight and goodbye to my dad for the week. This was unfamiliar territory for us; it was uncomfortable and raw and it didn't feel like us. Even though if felt so wrong, I knew there was nothing I could do about it.

I still held out hope, though. They were only separating, which meant that they would spend some time apart, and then realize that they couldn't live without each other. They would one day run back into each other's arms, with Endless Love playing in the background. Maybe there would be a white stallion in the background too. Then we would all go sing Edelweiss before escaping the Nazis in the lush hills of Austria.

Imagine my surprise when this didn't happen.

The weeks passed, and we got used to the routine of seeing my dad on the weekends, and being without him during the week. I started to tell my close friends that my parents had separated. It was something that I wasn't quite prepared to tell people. I never thought that our family would go through this.

The summer passed, and I prepared to go to college at Penn State University. My dad still hadn't moved back in. It seemed that the trial period was turning into a more permanent arrangement. In fact, he was looking for a house for himself. Heather had just graduated college and Kelly was out in the working world. Everyone was scattering.

By the time I left for college, it was clear that there would be no reconciliation. This was for good. During the separation, they didn't long for each other. The weekend reunions were not joyful. They were forced and awkward. It also became painfully clear to me that my parents were waiting for me to turn 18 to get a divorce. This had been brewing for a while, unbeknownst to me. There had been signs, I'm sure, but I certainly wasn't looking for them. If I had ever noticed anything, I put it in my file labeled "Nope, nope, everything's fine." But alas, this was happening and I couldn't deny it anymore.

This realization left me heartbroken. The thought of my parents not being together and our family getting used to a new life was terrifying and upsetting. Where would my dad live? Would my mom be okay in the house by herself now? Would their relationship always be contentious?

My home base was changing drastically and I was about to embark on a whole new journey, full of even more unknowns. I was heading to this new chapter of my life on rocky ground. In the fall, we piled into two separate cars and drove to Penn State. Amid a flurry of students, parents, minivans, and futons, we found our way to my dorm and got me settled in. I met Eileen, my roommate, in our closet-sized room. We were just two of thousands of nervous freshman, tiptoeing out of the nest into the world.

We spent the day picking up the essentials. The most important stop was the campus poster sale. Of the thousands of choices, I thoughtfully picked out a Dave Matthews poster and another one with a baby dressed up like a flower. Our next stop was at a boutique on College Avenue to pick out a wall tapestry, some incense and some candles. Strings of Christmas lights and funky lamps completed our college chic decor. Now that my dorm room looked like the inside of a rusty VW van parked at a Grateful Dead concert, I was all set.

We grabbed a quick bite to eat and then they left me. In college. By myself.

The nerve.

I felt, in a word, terrified. This was supposed to be the most exciting year of my life, and I was just scared shitless. How would I fit my HIV life into my college life? What if my class schedule interfered with my medicine schedule? What if people found out and they freaked out? What if I couldn't remember where any of my classes were? And what was home going to be like now?

Classes turned out to be the easy part of college life. I made friends in class and hung out with some of my roommate's friends whom she knew from high school. I went to parties. I went to football games. I did homework outside on the lawn. I drank too much Malibu rum and blue Hawaii, and threw up every 10 feet on the walk home. I acclimated.

I knew I had to tell my roommate Eileen that I was HIV positive. I was still on IL-2, which required that I give myself injections twice a day for a week, every eight weeks. Not really something I could hide from her. I told her one day after class, and thankfully, she was completely supportive. Little by little, it was becoming easier to tell people my story.

When it was IL-2 week, I knew I would get hit hard with those flu-like side effects. I tried to get my classwork done early in the week, knowing that I would be toast by mid-week. By Thursday, I was in bed day and night, trying to get past the fevers, chills, and aches.

One Friday night I was snuggled in bed. Eileen was at the mirror, getting ready to go out. I had told her that I would be sick that week because of the medicine.

"Are you sure you're okay?" she asked.

"Yeah, I'm okay. This is normal, I just have to wait it out."

She walked over to me and felt my forehead.

"Oh my God, you're burning up."

"I know. I'm okay though."

"Do you want me to stay here with you?"

"No! Go out, I'll be fine. I'm just going to watch a movie and go to sleep."

"Okay, are you sure?"

"Yeah, yeah, I'm sure."

"Okay, Sweetie, well, I'll be back later."

"Have fun," I said, and dozed off to sleep.

Those IL-2 days were miserable, but I was hopeful the drug was working against the virus.

Meanwhile, my parents made several visits during those first few months. They came on separate weekends. It was so strange to see them apart. Until that point in our lives, they were kind of a two-for-one deal, like most married parents. No so anymore. This one-on-one time introduced a whole new dynamic in our lives: hanging out with my dad, just the two of us.

My dad and I had always had the best relationship. I couldn't ask for a better dad, and I always used to joke with my sisters that I was his favorite. I always stuck by his side when he got home from work, and sat with him in his big, brown leather chair, watching westerns, or "shoot-'em-ups" as he called them. But that was in the context of a busy house with the rest of my family. Now it was just us on those weekends. This was new for us. I wasn't used to seeing my dad without my mom.

We figured it out, but not without some awkward growing pains. We were all trying to get used to our new lives. My mom, now in a house all by herself. My dad, in a brand new house all by himself. Heather and Kelly, acclimating to our parents' divorce as adults themselves. And me, in college, with two separate home bases.

On the weekends that they didn't visit, I drove home. I was still trying to find my place in college, and I ended up needed the comforts of home more than anything else. The problem was that the comforts of home were all different now. My dad had a house of his own. Even though I wanted to see my dad, I avoided going to his house because it was too much of a tangible representation of my parents' divorce. At that point, I felt like my security was out the window and that my world was coming down around me. My secure base had crumbled in two.

So I did what any college girl would have done. I stopped eating.

The notion of watching what I ate was completely foreign to me. Everyone around me seemed to be so concerned about what they ate, though. They constantly talked about food and trying to cut back on calories. At first I thought they were crazy. Then I thought I was crazy for not worrying about my weight too. I had always been able to eat like a tank and not gain weight, but I was in college now, so I had to start dieting. Right?

I carefully watched my friends' eating habits in the dining hall.

"You should always eat your salad first. You fill up on the low calorie stuff, then you don't eat as much other food."

"One time," one girl said proudly, "I trained myself to diet so much that one piece of pizza made my stomach hurt."

"This fro-yo is amazing, and it's fat-free. I'm just going to have this for dinner tonight."

I listened to them all and made mental notes.

I opted for fat-free everything. I skipped meals. I kept myself busy all day so that I would forget to eat. One day, I managed to go the whole day, only eating one half of a Pop-Tart.

I was hungry and miserable. I felt empty—literally and figuratively—but I was in control, finally.

The first time I went to NIH after I left for college, I hadn't dropped that much weight. It was nothing to be alarmed about. I didn't tell anyone there that I had decided to give up eating like a bad habit. No one needed to know. They just needed to see if the IL-2 was working. My preliminary lab results showed no improvement in my numbers from the IL-2. It was discouraging, but it wasn't hopeless yet. They wanted me to stay on it a few more months to see if it started working.

In the winter of my freshman year, I drove to camp for a reunion weekend. I was so thrilled to be going back to a place where everything was okay. It was literally an escape from my freshman year, which was turning into the year from hell. After the long seven-hour drive, I pulled into my happy place once again.

I greeted friends with warm embraces.

"You look so good!" everyone was telling me.

This is great, I thought, all this dieting is paying off.

We hung out that weekend, riding snow mobiles around the snow-covered camp and roasting s'mores in the dining hall fireplace.

My dear friend Lorrie and I were sitting on the couch in the dining hall, catching up.

"So how are you really doing?" she asked.

"Well, my life sucks right now. My parents are getting a divorce and college is weird. Half the time I love it and half the time I just want to go home."

"I'm worried about you, Jamie. You are so skinny."

I didn't say anything.

"What's been going on?" Lorrie pressed.

"I don't know. It's just easier not to eat. I'm fine though."

"You're not fine. You look terrible."

"But then why does everyone say I look great?" I was truly perplexed by this. Everyone did say I looked great.

"Because no one wants to tell you that you look like shit."

I didn't know what to say. She was absolutely right, and she was the only one who was able to tell me the truth.

I started to cry, and she snuggled me in for a hug.

"You have to talk to somebody about this."

"I do?"

"Yes. Promise me that when you get back to school, you will start seeing a counselor."

Through tears, I replied, "Okay, I promise."

I drove away from that cathartic weekend heavy-hearted. Intellectually, I knew Lorrie was right. But it wasn't like flipping a switch. Everyone around me was like this, so how was I supposed to be the only one to change?

The next month I went back to NIH for some repeat labs. I couldn't hide my weight loss from them any more, having dropped about 20 pounds from my already-thin frame. They were very concerned, but they immediately assumed that it was just related to the IL-2 not working. My labs confirmed that the IL-2 was, in fact, not working at all. My numbers were not improving at all. The IL-2 was taking more of a toll on my body than it was on the virus.

I confided in my trusted counselor, Lori, that I had stopped eating. I was still skirting around the word "anorexic" with quaint euphemisms, but I really did know what was going on. And I knew that I had to nip it in the bud.

It didn't take long for reality to set in, and for me to understand that I was killing myself. The benefit of being a professional patient my whole life was that I couldn't really smoke anything by anybody. I had to get my shit together.

Back at school, I went to the campus health center and signed up to work with a free counselor. I was committed to turning this around. I had absolutely no choice, because I was about to start a new drug protocol that had to be taken with a high calorie diet. Slowly, I taught myself to eat normally again. This was no easy process, and it wasn't an overnight change, but I did get out of those habits.

Which made being around my friends even harder. They had no idea I had become anorexic, and I think they were so focused on their own self-images that they didn't notice that I had wasted away and then put the weight back on. Now, when they gave their unsolicited dieting advice, I looked at them with disdain.

Do you know what you are doing to people? And to yourselves? I thought.

It became harder to hang out with them. As the months of my second semester passed, I was slowly drifting away from their group.

I started my next drug protocol during the second semester of freshman year. This one, Ritonovir, didn't involve injections, thankfully. It did however require the consumption of a high calorie diet. I went from starving myself in an effort to control my world to packing in the calories however I could get them. If I didn't take the Ritonovir with high-caloric foods, I got a wicked stomach ache.

I carried around a lunch bag full of donuts and 600-calorie supplement shakes. I had about five minutes between classes to choke down a thick chocolate shake and two donuts with my afternoon meds. When I got it all down, I schlepped into my Eastern Philosophy class, feeling like a bloated cow.

This routine was exhausting but I kept it up for several months. Multiple trips back to NIH for labs revealed that my numbers still weren't coming up. This drug didn't like me any more than I liked it, and we parted ways.

I finished out freshman year on yet another medication, and luckily, I responded well. My numbers got better and the side effects were minimal. It seemed that I had found a sweet spot after many months of trial and error.

I was beginning to find a sweet spot with my parents' divorce, as well. The individual visits became less awkward. We were all coming to terms with what life looked like now. My mom and dad were thriving in their separate lives, and they got to a point where they could be cordial and even friendly with each other during family events and holidays.

As freshman year ended, I drove away from my dorm without looking back at the tumultuous year that I was leaving. College brought with it new challenges and some unexpected monsters, and I was ready to move on.

CHAPTER THIRTEEN

DATING. Ugh. Let me just say one thing about dating. Under the most normal circumstances, dating is painful. There are those people out there who love dating. It's like an amateur sport that they are very good at. I don't understand those people. I give them all the credit in the world, but I don't understand them. It's like people who run because it "makes them feel alive." Really?

I think my awkward adolescent years really stuck with me, because I approached dating with a certain level of anxiety. Always in my head was a nagging fear that I would do something wrong to screw things up. Like not knowing everything about sports, or being too clingy, or having some sort of terminal disease. Oh wait . . .

Don't get me wrong, that spark of attraction is electrifying. It can put you on cloud nine and make you impervious to the monotony of everyday life. You are in an annoyingly good mood, to the point that those around you want to punch you in the face. Suddenly the long line at Starbucks isn't irritating—it's a great occasion to chat with perfect strangers. Getting pulled over? Yes please! What a great opportunity to thank a police officer for his service. Getting mugged? Excellent! I was just thinking of how I could contribute more to my community!

That feeling of bliss is exhilarating and I loved basking in it as much as the next girl. But once I got past the initial excitement over a potential love connection, I started to think about all the details. Starting small, the first question was, what should I wear? This was not a simple "what matches what" situation. It's a very complicated formula, involving the setting of the date, day of the week, weather, time of day, current menstrual cycle location, and some astrological factor to determine the optimal date outfit. There should be an app for that. The goal is to feel comfortable, yet stunningly attractive and effortlessly flawless. No big thing.

Once I'm perfectly coiffed, dressed, and accessorized (and now in real need of a nap), the actual date begins. Do I meet him there? Does he pick me up? Do I pick him up? (No.) I want to come off as independent but needy enough to make him feel useful and manly. Plus, what if he turns out to be a psychopath? It's always best if psychopaths don't know where you live. Write that down.

We are finally on the date. Now, do I order a drink, or do I wait until he does? I don't want to come off like

Drunky McGee, but I also don't want him to think that I am uptight. Then if I do order a drink, what do I get? Beer, the I'm-the-kind-of-girl-you-can-relax-around-your-buddies-with drink? Wine, the I'm-a-mature-adult-who-can-handle-her-business drink? Fruity cocktail? No, too fruity. Hard cocktail? No, too serious. Shots? Not so much.

We haven't even gotten to the appetizers yet, and I'm exhausted.

What was really looming in the back of my head was the "There's something I need to tell you" conversation. When I went on first dates, I tried to focus on enjoying the moment and relaxing, but I had this ISSUE looming. It's like a piece of a popcorn kernel that gets lodged between your teeth. You can go on with your day just fine, but it's really annoying. I would always be slightly distracted by this, which prevented me from fully opening up.

Being HIV positive made me look at every guy I met through the "Could you withstand THE TALK?" lens. Although this was a very annoying thought to have while experiencing the initial spark of attraction, it served as a very good litmus test of boyfriend potential. It weeded out a bunch of goobers, that's for sure. For me, it ranks up there with spiritual beliefs, political leanings, and favorite movie. All of those can be deal-makers or breakers—especially the movie one. So, with every potentially serious guy I met, I was going through the conversation in my head and thinking, *how is he going to handle this?* There were some guys with whom it was an easy decision to tell or not tell, and therefore, to pursue or not pursue. With some guys it didn't take much conversation to realize that this kind of information would be the fastest and most efficient way to send them running for the hills. But honestly, most guys passed the test of being tellable.

Next was the question of when to tell them. I'm sure there is a split-second window of time when the time is right to tell a romantic interest that you are HIV positive. It has to be after enough time has passed to be comfortable enough to have a serious conversation. But it can't be too far into a relationship that the other person feels you have been holding out on them. For me, this was looming over my head with every potential relationship, so I opted to tell people sooner rather than later. I couldn't bear getting too attached, with this big IF hanging out there.

I was surprised to learn that most guys took it surprisingly well. In college, I began dating Mark, a guy I knew from high school. Ironically, he lived on my street and it wasn't until we were attending a school of 50,000 people that we found each other. Mark was a year older than me, but I assumed he had heard about my big announcement, as he was friends with people in my graduating class.

Could it be? Could I actually go into a relationship without having to have The Talk? Well, that would be just lovely. We went on a few dates, saw *The Nutcracker* on campus, went swing dancing together. Apparently, I was very cultured (and 80 years old) when I was in college. Everything was going swimmingly, but I didn't know for sure that he knew.

There was only one way to find out: call him from a pay phone as an anonymous surveyor and ask if he knew anyone who was HIV positive. Hey, I guess there were two ways to find out. The pay phone stunt would have been good, but I opted for the old-fashioned way.

We were in my dorm room one night, canoodling on my futon — probably watching Dawson's Creek — and I said to him, "Hey, I kind of have to talk to you about something."

"About what?"

"Well, there's something about me that I'm not sure you know."

"Okayyyyy."

"I'm HIV positive."

I wasn't beating around the bush with this one. I honestly thought he already knew, and that I would be saved from telling the whole drawn-out story.

"I didn't know that."

"Oh."

Apparently small towns aren't as gossipy as I thought.

"Well," I continued, "Yeah. I am. I have been since I was three. I had a heart defect and had to have open heart surgery. They gave me a blood transfusion, and it was infected with HIV."

He was quiet. Nodding. And he started to snuggle me more. This is great, I was thinking. He was taking this really well.

"I'm really healthy. I take meds and I have to go to the doctor every few months in DC, but I've always been really healthy. I wasn't sure if you knew, because

I kind of made an announcement to the school when I graduated."

Finally he spoke. "Yeah, actually, maybe I did know. I think I remember someone telling me that, now that I think about it."

What?! Seriously? Maybe this is egocentric of me, but isn't that something you don't really forget? I mean, it's not like, "Oh, I forgot that you were allergic to shellfish, or hate roses." This was kind of a big deal, no?

Nonetheless, he knew now, and we could move on. I assumed that because we had known each other in high school, and that he knew, we would stick together, get matching tattoos, and wander off into the sunset with each other. I thought this relationship was too big to fail. Well, we all know how that turned out for the banks.

I naively expected him to be completely okay with it, but as it turned out, he had a lot of thinking to do. I was shocked that he had to ponder this, and I started panicking. This was not what I had planned. No! We had so much going for us!

After a day or so, I called him to see how he was doing. I wanted to talk. I wanted to see where he was. He said that he couldn't get together because he was hanging out with his buddies. Yeah, I didn't care. I told him that I really needed to talk and begged him to come over.

He did agree to come over. He cared enough for me to leave his buddies to talk, so I had high hopes. We met in the common room of my dorm and sat down on the overstuffed sofa. The students around us were doing homework over lattes, and we started to talk about HIV.

"I'm so glad you came over. I just need to know how you are feeling about everything."

"Yeah."

I waited. Waited for him to say, "I've thought a lot about this, and I love you. We can deal with this together."

But all I got was silence.

I tried to get the conversation going.

"So I know you were shocked by what I told you. I really thought you already knew."

He put his arm around me, which I took as a good sign. But still, no words.

"I know this is a lot to think about, and I don't know what I would do if I were in your shoes. I can't ask anyone to choose to deal with this."

"I know," he said.

We looked at each other and I was desperately waiting to hear those reassuring words.

"So what are we going to do?" I asked. I had to put it out there. No more screwing around.

"Well. I care about you so much. I just don't know if this is something that I can deal with," he finally said.

Now it was my turn to be quiet.

"I want you to be healthy and happy and I want to know that you're okay. But I don't think I can handle it."

I nodded. "I understand," I said, "I wouldn't ask you to do anything that you're not comfortable with."

We sat up straight, and he rubbed my arm.

"Well, I'm glad you told me. It makes me sad, but I don't know that I would do the same thing if the roles were reversed."

I had no other words to say. All I could think about at this point was keeping it together in the middle of that common room. We hugged and went our separate ways.

I went back to my hall and knocked on the door of my good friend, Kristy, who lived across the hall. When she opened the door, I looked at her and burst into tears. Kristy knew my story, and I knew I could be myself around her.

"Oh my God! What happened?"

She pulled me inside her room and sat me down on her bed, hugging me.

"What's going on?" she asked.

Between sobs, I managed to eke out, "Mark said he couldn't deal with it and we broke up."

"Oh, Jamie," she said.

I curled up in a ball and sobbed my eyes out. I couldn't speak. She didn't speak. She rubbed my back as I sobbed hysterically for what seemed like hours. I became more exhausted and winded with every heaving breath, and eventually passed out. It was all too much for me to deal with in that moment and my body literally just powered down. Moments later, I woke up and was able to sit up and take a deep breath.

This was the first big rejection I'd experienced, and I was not ready to deal with it. Was this what my life would be like? A series of great people, great first dates, then screeching halts? I didn't know where to go from there.

The only thing I could do was to go on with day-to-day life. My mom always told me, "This too shall pass," and I clung to that hope for dear life.

As the days and weeks passed, I began to reconcile my feelings about the break-up with Mark. Through it all, I bore no animosity toward him. It wasn't his fault. It just sucked.

College was no place to wallow in self-pity, and I focused on moving on and spending time with friends. I spent a lot time with my friend Jenn. She and I lived on the same hallway and became buddies at the beginning of the year. We went to the dining hall together, and every Wednesday, we gathered with the rest of the dorm girls to watch Dawson's Creek which, by the way, was a staple of my college years, and pretty much the best show ever about teen angst. Jenn and I bonded over health issues because she had a chronic condition as well. We swapped stories about taking meds and going to doctor's appointments. I felt comfortable confiding in her, so I told her that I was HIV positive.

Jenn's friend Dan also spent time with us. Dan and I were friends, with an undertone of flirtation to our relationship. I had a crush on Dan and suspected that the feeling was mutual. Our attraction manifested itself in a few make-out sessions, but nothing more. Just good clean college fun. Toward the end of the year, Dan seemed to lose interest in me, and our relationship shifted from flirt-fest to just friends. This is not entirely uncommon for college; let's face it, guys and girls in college have the attention spans of a gnat when it comes to romantic relationships. I didn't think much of it, until . . .

It was the last week of school and all the students were wrapping up finals, packing up dorm rooms, and saying goodbyes. Dan and I were in my dorm room, saying goodbye for the summer. He gave me a big hug and said, "Promise me that you'll take care of yourself." What?! Since when did hormone-fueled college boys become ultra-nurturing? Since never, that's when.

This wasn't a casual "take care" sentiment. This was a statement rooted in genuine concern for my well-being. I knew something was up. I knew that he knew. But I hadn't told him, so how did he know? In that moment, I was thrown off-guard and I didn't say anything. I replied with an awkward, "Okayyyyyyy," and we went on with our goodbyes.

He left me confused—very touched, but confused nonetheless. There was really only one person who could have told him. Only one mutual friend who knew about me. And wait a minute. This person happened to have a monster crush on Dan. A bigger crush than I did, for certain. Like, a restraining order-in-the-making crush. Only one person: Jenn.

Not one to fester and speculate, I decided to confront her. When Dan left, I walked across the hall and two doors down to Jenn's room. She was packing dishes into a white plastic crate.

"Hey, Jenn."

"Hey."

"I can't believe it's the end of the year and we're leaving."

"I know, it's crazy."

"So, I was just with Dan."

Silence.   Eye contact ceased and desisted. Suspicions confirmed.

I said, "He said something kind of weird to me. He said, 'Promise me that you'll take care of yourself.' Isn't that weird?"

I figured I'd give her one chance to 'fess up.

"That is weird," she said. Fail.

"Why would he say that?" I asked, feigning ignorance.

"I don't know," she said, feigning innocence.

"Does he know about me?"

"I don't know. He might, but I don't know."

"How would he know?"

Silence.

"Well, did you tell him something?" I pressed on.

"Well, he asked me one day why you take medicine, so I guess I told him."

Son of a.....

"Well, it really wasn't your place to tell him. I don't really care that he knows, but I should have been the one to tell him, not you."

"I was just answering his question. I didn't think it was a big deal."

Yeah right.

Not wanting to drag things out, I just said, "Well, whatever. Have a nice summer." There was no need to get into a big argument over a done deal. We were all going our separate ways anyway. I figured that she felt guilty enough as it was, and there wasn't any point in lecturing her on the importance of being a trustworthy person.

Needless to say, we didn't reconnect when the next school year began.

Luckily this only happened once that I was aware of. What made it hard was that I had no control over how my status was disclosed. Deciding to tell someone my status was a big deal, and not a decision that I ever took lightly. When I did make that decision, I gave them my background, explained the details, and answered their questions. I planned it out. I led the conversation. I had control. This kind of personal disclosure put me in a place of acute vulnerability and subjected me to whatever kind of reaction the other person might have. Being able to tell people myself gave me some sense of autonomy over the situation. I never had a choice about getting HIV, but I could choose who I told and how I told them. When that was taken away, it left me feeling naked and powerless.

Luckily, heartache and backstabbing were speed bumps and not the norm for me. The good times far outweighed the bad, and college continued to be a blast. At the end of my sophomore year I met two of my best friends in the world, Morgan and Tricia. We had lived on the same hall the entire year and hadn't hung out until about two weeks before the semester ended. We went to see *Never Been Kissed* with Drew Barrymore (Drew wasn't with us, she was just in the movie . . .), and we have been cosmically inseparable ever since.

Morgan, Tricia and I made a career out of getting dolled-up and going out on the town to frat parties. We were so cool. Each Halloween, we dressed as some sort of sexy trio—Fly Girls, Charlie's Angels, basically anything that allowed us to dress up like sluts and do the Charlie's Angels pose. Even the purest of girls are allowed to do that on Halloween. Everyone knows that.

Many of our ensembles, Halloween or otherwise, required a bare midriff. Which, of course, required tanning. In preparation for our weekend of parties, we had a nightly routine of slathering Neutrogena tanning lotion all over our stomachs. Then we would lie down on the dorm room floor, watching TV as it dried. It had a very pungent smell to it, but we endured. We were very dedicated to this routine.

This problem with this plan is that we didn't bother to tan the rest of our pasty little bodies. The result? Three orange Creamsicles with white arms, faces, and legs, and orange stripes on our stomachs. And we smelled.

But if you asked us, we were hot stuff. So the three Creamsicles hit the town every weekend, meeting friends at our favorite fraternity houses. We danced like it was our job. We met boys, we let loose, and we just had a blast.

And this is where I always had to keep myself in check. I knew that I couldn't go out and sleep with a bunch of guys in college, because I had this big secret. Sure, I could have, but it just would have made me feel deceptive. And icky. I couldn't let loose with this hanging over my head. So while I still had the time of my life, I knew that I had limits. Meanwhile, I watched a lot of fellow party people make boneheaded decisions in a drunken stupor. At times, I really resented how careless people could be. They thought they were invincible. I was stuck with being HIV positive. They had the power to protect themselves, but they were still being idiots.

That said, I can't say that I was a saint, or that I went through college standing on my soapbox. I had the time of my life. Even though I was always responsible, I still made a fool of myself in a drunken stupor—but hardly ever, Mom and Dad. It's best to stop talking about this now.

CHAPTER FOURTEEN

SOME days you wake up and you have no idea that your life is about to change. That's what Tuesday, July 5, 2005 was for me. By this time I had graduated college, completed a child life internship, and gotten a job in Northern Virginia. Little Jamie was all grown up. That Tuesday morning I woke up, went to work, and planned to meet my friends for happy hour at our favorite Tex-Mex cantina right by the hospital. I showed up after a long uneventful day at work, ready to relax and enjoy some $2 margaritas. Those would be the best $14 I ever spent.

I walked inside and scanned the bar for my friends, who were seated at a bar table, a couple of drinks in already. I walked up to our table and saw someone there whom I didn't recognize. Who was this guy, busting in on our happy hour? Suddenly the situation changed from "casual happy hour with friends" to "casual happy hour with friends, and oh by the way, I should also try to be cute and charming." The empty seat also happened to be next to him. I sat down and my friend Kerri introduced me to the mystery man, Paul, who was her neighbor. Nice to meet you. Where's my margarita?

I pulled the typical uninterested-girl routine, and didn't really talk to Paul for the first half-hour or so. I was playing that game I hated, being a jerk because I was interested.

Finally, after a few fishbowl-sized margaritas, I turned to Paul and asked, "So, what do you do?"

"I'm a teacher."

"Really? What do you teach?"

"Third grade."

"That's cool," I said, "I always wanted to be a teacher because I love writing on chalk boards." That wasn't a line; it was the honest truth.

He laughed. "Yeah, it's pretty cool. What do you do?"

"I'm a child life specialist."

He gave me a puzzled look that everyone gives me when I tell them that.

"You don't know what that is, do you?" I asked.

"Nope."

"I work with kids in the hospital who are getting radiology procedures. I help them understand what's going on and help them through their procedures. My job is basically to help lower their anxiety when they come into the hospital so they can cope better with what's happening."

Soon enough, we weren't talking to anyone else at

the table but each other.

"So what kind of music do you like to listen to?" he asked.

"I like pretty much everything except for country."

"Do you like Dave Matthews?"

"Um, Dave Matthews is my favorite band. I love him."

"Are you serious? You do?" he asked.

Oh great, I thought, this is one of those guys who hates Dave Matthews because he's too college-y or too popular. Whatever. I though he was going to be cool, but forget it. If he's about to bust on Dave Matthews for being a sell-out, then this is over.

"Dave Matthews is awesome," he said. "Nobody realizes how good he really is. What's your favorite DMB song?"

"Well, I have a lot, but Proudest Monkey is up there."

"Nice."

"Mmm hmmmm," I said, smiling like a goober.

"So if you want to, I could show you my chalkboard in my classroom. You could write all over it." Smooth.

"Okay!" I said, "that would be amazing. I could live out my childhood dreams."

"But you'd have to give me your number if you wanted to set up some private chalkboard time."

"Well then, I guess I'll have to give it to you." I grabbed a napkin and wrote my full name and number on it for him, completely abandoning the uninterested-girl routine.

"See, I have really good handwriting," I said as I

handed him the napkin.

"It's really good. I'm impressed."

That's right he was.

We left the bar and I drove home thinking, Hmmm...I think I really like this boy. I wonder if I'll ever hear from him again.

And then the most amazing thing happened. He called. The next day. Anyone who has ever been on the social scene knows how rare this is. It's like finding a box of puppies and cash on the sidewalk. It rarely happens, but when it does, how much fun?!

We went on our first date that Friday. Paul picked me up and on our way to dinner, he said, "I have something for you."

"Really?" I said. "I love presents."

"It's in the glove compartment."

Okay, this either could have been the beginning of a beautiful love story or a psycho slasher movie; who knew what was in that glove box?! I opened it up and there was a fresh box of colored chalk just for me. It was pretty much the best gift I have ever gotten. A present on our first date? I liked this boy.

We went to dinner at Harry's Tap Room in Arlington, Virginia, followed by a walk around the city and cocktails at Bertucci's. We talked about everything . . . well, almost everything. I still had THE TALK lingering in the back of my mind, but mostly I was just enjoying our time together. By the end of the night, I was a smitten kitten. When it ended, we made no bones about planning to see each other again. None of this playing coy nonsense—we liked each other and we didn't care who knew it.

Approximately nine hours went by until we saw each other again. Our second date turned into an entire day of being together. We went to a crabfest together with a group of friends. Neither of us are huge fans of crabs, or all the effort that goes into picking them. We bonded over watching all the weirdos eat crabs while we drank beer and ate hot dogs. I know I'm betraying my Maryland routes by admitting this, but I can't help it. I'm very lazy and the thought of working that hard for my food makes me lose my appetite. Plus, those suckers look like they could bite you back at any given moment. Your food shouldn't scare you.

After the crabfest, we strolled around Reston Town Center and saw a movie, *Mr. and Mrs. Smith*. We finished our day with snuggling and canoodling at Paul's place.

Approximately another nine hours passed, bringing us to date number three. It was a Sunday, and we spent another day of fun together. By this time, we were both pretty smitten and realized that this was something special. I was beginning to feel that weight of the "untold part of me" getting heavier and heavier. With every moment we spent together, I thought, Is this going to be another moment that just turns into a bittersweet memory? This relationship was looking really good, but it hadn't faced the true test yet. With every perfect moment that we spent together, the untold truth was still hovering overhead. The time had come and we had to have The Talk.

We were sitting on Paul's balcony and it seemed a

good time to take another flying leap off the cliff and hope the parachute opened.

"So. There's something that you should know about me."

"Okaaaaay......" The eyebrows raised. Who knows what was going through his head: Is she going to tell me that she's married? She used to be a man? She's just using me for my access to chalkboards?

"It has to do with my health. It's something that I feel anyone I am close to should know about, and there's definitely something happening between you and me."

Nodding....

"When I was born, I had a congenital heart defect called Tetrology of Fallot. It basically meant that I had four large defects in my heart. I had surgery when I was three to repair it, which was a success."

"Wow," he said.

Oh, I'm not done, buddy, I thought. Just wait.

"During the surgery, I had to have a blood transfusion. This all happened in 1982 when they weren't screening blood products. It turns out that the blood transfusion I got was infected with HIV, so I am HIV positive."

Dramatic pause.

"I'm very healthy and I've been healthy my whole life. My family found out when I was eight and I found out when I was ten. I started taking medicine for it when I was 10 and it's been really well-controlled. I've been very lucky to be so healthy my whole life, and really the hardest part about it for me is telling people like this."

Paul, a very quiet and calm person by nature, hadn't budged since I started unloading this bombshell. He sat back in the chair, elbows on the armrest, chin resting on his index fingers. He nodded slowly, and I could see in his wide eyes that he was shocked. I also saw his eyes welling with tears.

"Wow," he said.

"I know. I don't feel right about getting close to people without telling them. I know this is a lot of information. You probably need time to process this. You can ask me any questions you have; when I tell people, I know there's a possibility that they may not want to deal with it."

At this thought, my eyes started to well with tears.

"I wouldn't ask anyone to choose to deal with this, and I can't blame anyone for choosing not to. I love being with you, but I understand if this is something that you don't want to deal with."

Paul took my hand. He said, "I think this is something that will be okay, but I need time to think."

I nodded, "It's in your court now; I'll just leave it up to you to call me if or when you want to talk about it."

As I drove home, I struggled with a mix of feelings. I was relieved that it was finally out in the open, but I was also terrified that it would end our relationship. There was a lot on the line with this one, and I had no idea what was going to happened from here.

Paul called me the next day. "What are you doing right now?" he asked.

"I'm driving home from my doctor's appointment."

"Will you be home soon?"

"Yeah."

"Can I come over."

"Yeah, for sure. I'll be there in about 10 minutes."

He came over and we sat on the couch in my little basement apartment. I could tell that he was still reeling. He had some questions, and I could tell that he had spent a significant chunk of the past 24 hours Googling away. I wasn't expecting that, and it actually kind of threw me off. I was expecting us to talk about me, but we were talking about HIV.

During that conversation, I could tell that Paul was in the information-gathering phase, and he hadn't quite come to the point of resolution. It was only 24 hours after our initial conversation, so it was still quite early on in the processing. We talked about my meds and what my life was like, living with HIV. Paul had a lot of questions. Questions that I didn't even know the answers to. He had put in a lot of time researching this.

This was all new to me, because I had ever spent this much time talking about HIV. I was kind of over it, to be honest. All I needed to know was whether or not Paul was going to leave me. But we just kept talking.

A few days went by and we checked in over the phone periodically. Those hours and days crept by at a snail's pace. I tried to distract myself from this big unknown, but I couldn't do it. I couldn't mentally or emotionally disconnect from the situation or Paul, and I found myself more stressed than I had ever been in past relationships during that waiting period. It was like emotional purgatory.

I called Heather during that week to tell her how things were going. "I told Paul on Sunday."

"How did it go?"

"He took it well, but now he is just researching the hell out of it. I don't know what he's thinking and it's making me crazy."

"You just gotta give him time, Jame. He's never had to deal with this before. If he ends up deciding that he can't deal with it, then he's not the guy for you anyway."

"I know, but I just can't disconnect from this guy. When I told other guys, I kind of checked out until they decided that it was okay. I can't do that with Paul. It's all I can think about and I'm going crazy. I have The Pit."

The Pit is this feeling you get in your chest when you are so terrified that you are going to lose something that is so precious. I was terrified that Paul would walk away. We had only known each other for a week, so he didn't have a lot invested in this. It wouldn't have taken much for him to just walk away.

Days passed, and we got together again for more talking. I was a stress monkey—I just needed to know what he was going to do.

We sat down on my couch again.

"So, I think this is going to be okay," he said.

"You do?"

"Yeah. I mean, it's definitely not something I was expecting, but we can deal with it."

"It makes me so happy to hear you say that. I have been going crazy. I know we've only known each other for a few days, but I love being with you. I haven't really felt like this before."

"Yeah, I'm feeling some pretty strong feelings here."

I could finally breathe a sigh of relief. Paul was in this with me. He had no plans to bail.

We also secretly realized at this point that this relationship was for keeps. It was an amazing evolution of vulnerability, doubt, anguish, acceptance and pure happiness. Once we realized where we were headed, it was full speed ahead.

Paul quickly became the perfect boyfriend, advocate, and supporter-extraordinaire. He came with me to all my doctor's appointments, met with my doctor, asked questions, and willingly accepted this into his life. It became a "nobody puts Baby in a corner" scenario with Paul as my great protector. I was thrilled, touched, and slightly freaked out that he now knew more about HIV than I did. He was teaching me things that I never knew about—the nerve! Thank God Google is free, because otherwise we'd be broke. Highly educated, but broke.

I couldn't have asked for a better supporter. Without hesitation or any hint of complaint, Paul accepted this and everything it meant for him. Obviously, it had an impact on our sexual relationship. Welcome to the world of barrier protection, friends. And you thought condoms were just for college kids. This was only one of the aspects of his life that suddenly changed, and he accepted it willingly.

Paul and I were fairly inseparable by this point. Every day, at the end of the work day, we were together. When the weekend rolled around, we were together. We didn't even have to be doing anything; we just wanted to be together.

Two months after we started dating, Paul and I went out to dinner at McCormick and Schmick's, one of our favorite restaurants. We sat down and Paul ordered a bottle of champagne.

"Ooo, champagne?" I said.

"We're celebrating," he said.

"What are we celebrating?"

"Just us," he said.

After dinner, we walked around Reston Town Center in the balmy summer weather.

Paul said, "Do you want a coffee or anything?"

"No, I'm good, but you can get something if you want."

"Yeah, I want something. Let's go into Starbucks."

Paul ordered a dopio—two straight shots of espresso. I looked at him with the "what's wrong with you?" one-eyebrow lift.

"Are you okay?" I asked.

"Yeah, why?"

"I don't know. You just seem anxious. And you're drinking a double shot of espresso at 9pm."

"Oh. Do I seem anxious?"

"Mm hmmm."

"Oh. I'm fine. Ready to go home?"

"Okay." (weirdo......)

We went home and I went into the bathroom. A minute later, I walked out to candles, roses, and champagne sitting on the coffee table.

"Oh my God," I said, and I started to feel giddy.

Paul just smiled. "Come over here. Sit down."

I sat down on the black leather chair. Paul knelt down and said, "Baby, I love you so much. Will you marry me?" And he pulled out the most beautiful ring on the planet.

"Yes!" It was all I could get out. I was delirious. This was one of the most amazing moments of my life. There were times in my life when I didn't know if I would live to see adulthood, and if so, if I would find someone whom I loved who would also be willing to deal with all of me. And it was all happening.

"We're getting married!" I finally yelled, when I got my words back. I was fairly certain that Paul already knew that, but it needed to be said, and said loudly. "I have to call my mom!" I said next.

"She already knows," Paul told me.

Paul had Googled my mom to find her work number, tracked her down and asked for her permission to ask me to marry him. He did the same with my dad. This floored me. We had already established ourselves as a fairly non-traditional couple, but for some reason, this step of asking for permission really touched me. It also confirmed to me how serious this was. It wasn't a compulsive decision for either of us. It was for real.

The next few days were spent sharing the good news with friends and family. Most were shocked that we were engaged after only two months. Many of my extended family members didn't even know I had a boyfriend, so the engagement news was particularly shocking. Those conversations went something along these lines:

"I have some great news."

"What?"

"I'm getting married!"

"Really? Congratulations! We didn't even know you were dating anyone. Are you pregnant?"

Ha.

After we told everyone that we were getting married, and that I was not in fact pregnant, we got to planning. The first order of business was to pick out my dress. This is the moment I had been waiting for my whole life, not because it was a symbolic representation of my survival; but because wedding dresses are amazing. Seriously. When else can you dress up like a princess and have people ooooh and ahhhhh over you?

Oh right, beauty pageants.

Okay, but besides that, when?

It's an amazing perk to an already-euphoric feeling, and I was ready to go. With a group of girlfriends in tow, I drove to a bridal store, giddy with excitement. The doors opened and a choir of angels started singing, as I scanned the sea of white and ivory laid out before me like clouds. Belinda Carlisle was right; Heaven is a place on earth, and it was located in a Northern Virginia strip mall.

"Welcome! Come in!" the employees said.

Please God, don't recognize me from the time I came in here last year and tried on dresses with my friend, I prayed. It was a moment of weakness. Every girl gets at least one.

"Who's the bride?"

"I am," I said. (This time for real!)

"Do you know what you are looking for?"

"Yes. I'm looking for something strapless, maybe a sweetheart neckline, beaded on top, kind of princess-y but not too poofy, with a long bodice and a medium-length train . . . I mean, just off the top of my head."

She gave her co-worker a sly look and said, "I think I have just the dress for you."

She took me to a rack of dresses and pulled one out to show me. I looked at that dress and fell in love for the second time in as many months.

"I love this!" I said.

"This is a beautiful dress and it has everything you described."

"Okay, yes, I want to try that on. Where is your dressing room?"

"You should pick out a few other dresses to try on too," they advised.

"Okay, I can do that." I figured I might as well do that while I was there.

I picked out a few others and went into the dressing room, eyes on the prize on that first dress. Like an astronaut, I climbed into it and got zipped up with the help of a team of experts. I walked out and stepped up on the pedestal to take a look. And then I reached the point of maximum cheesiness, and cried. It was official: I was a blubbering mess, and I had found my dress.

The best part—it was just comfortable enough to serve as a special party or vacuuming dress after the wedding. There is nothing wrong with that. That dress has paid for itself tenfold by now.

Now that I had the two most important details in the bag, the guy and the dress, I continued on with wedding planning. Paul and I drove all over Northern Virginia and DC, looking for the perfect spot for our wedding. We locked in the venue, the caterer, the florist, the photographer—all the essentials. The big day was only months away.

Throughout this planning process, I periodically stepped back and basked in this joy of finding my match, and planning our lives together. This is something I didn't know would ever happen. This is what "normal" people do, and I was actually getting to do it.

Four months before the wedding, I got what I thought was a bad case of food poisoning. It started off as a typical stomach bug, where my body wouldn't tolerate any food or liquids. I felt awful, but I knew it would pass. I just had to wait it out. After a couple of days, I decided I needed to go into the urgent care center to get IV fluids. I just couldn't keep anything down, and I knew that I would feel better if I could get rehydrated.

Paul took me to the urgent care center, stopping at every bathroom on the way. It was miserable, but I finally got settled in, with IV fluids on board. A few hours and a couple of doses of anti-nausea medication later, I felt slightly rejuvenated and ready to go home. They did blood work while I was there, just to make sure that everything was okay.

Back at home, I rested and tried to get liquids down,

to no avail. I wasn't getting better. Paul was a saint during this time. I was such a mess; I could barely move, much less clean up after myself, so Paul was left with that lovely task. He did it without complaint or one hint of being grossed out. He stayed home from work and tended to my every need.

The hospital called to tell me that my lab results were normal. I was relieved and frustrated at the same time. If they didn't find anything, then why was I still so sick? Four days into this and nothing was changing. My body was getting weaker and weaker, and I was starting to get worried. I usually bounced back from illnesses, but this was dragging on. We went back to urgent care for a second time. I felt like my body was shutting down and my only relief thus far had been IV fluids and anti-nausea meds.

They placed an IV, got my fluids running, and put me in a quiet room. I just lay there on an uncomfortable stretcher, getting frustrated with my lack of recovery. It was the first time in a very long time that I felt weak and helpless. I wondered if I was going to get over this. Here I had just gotten engaged and was planning my normal life, and it had come to a screeching halt. Was I going to die? I knew Paul was thinking the same thing. We hadn't even known each other for a year. When I told him about being HIV positive, I assured him that I had always been very healthy. Did he think now that I hadn't been honest with him? Was he going to regret taking this on? Was he going to get scared off, and run before we get married? What if I died? How would Paul tell his friends and family that his new fiancé died? Why did Paul have to go through this pain, for only a few months of being together?

I wallowed, which I don't normally do. I felt defeated. I felt like I had a glimpse into a normal life, and then someone smacked me in the face with reality. How stupid was I to think that I could lead a normal life? I didn't know what was going to happen, but I was worried. I could see the look of concern in Paul's face as he sat by my side. We were together in that room, neither of us knowing what would happen.

Hours passed and I finally turned a corner. A second set of labs revealed that I had rotovirus, a nasty gastrointestinal bug.

The first time I kept food down was a blessing, and I finally felt my strength coming back. I was feeling like myself again, and not a sick person. My favorite feeling in the world, relief, returned to me. I was back on track with my life plans. This wasn't the end and I was still strong.

We got married on a gorgeous and perfect spring day in April. My mom and dad walked me down the aisle. I looked ahead and saw Paul there waiting for me. This was the moment I had been waiting for. I was about to start a life with my perfect match. I wanted that moment to last forever. (I should have picked a venue with a longer aisle.) Step by step, I got closer to him, and my emotions took over during those last few steps, which is precisely why I don't have any pictures of that part. I was tearing up but trying so hard not to start sobbing like a blubbering bride. I'm not a cute crier, so

I'm sure I looked like I had just gotten punched or something, with my face all scrunched up, trying to hold back the tears. I intentionally didn't wear my veil over my face, because I thought it was a rather antiquated—and even insulting—tradition. Looking back, I would do it differently. Screw women's lib. I should have covered that mess.

When I reached Paul, I forgot to give my parents a hug and a kiss. I just left them in the dust and went right up to Paul. Composed and ready, we read our vows to each other in a short but sweet ceremony, in the afternoon sun. The rest of the evening was a dream, relaxed and free of formality, and just what we wanted. No garter toss, eww. My dad does not need to see my new husband going up my dress like a maniac. No bouquet toss. Really? It's like tossing a prime rib into an alligator pit. There will be blood.

We danced our first dance to Dave Matthews Band's "I'll Back You Up." Dave (because we are on a first name basis, don't you know) sings,

Do what you will, always
Walk where you like, your steps
Do as you please, I'll back you up

That's what life with Paul has been like since the day I met him. We back each other up, no matter what. I have been blessed to have an amazing family in my corner my whole life. When things got tough, they were there, every step of the way, without fail. And now, I had that in a whole other dimension. What I found in Paul was someone who willingly took on everything that my life brought with it. For me, it meant that Paul thought about what his life would be like with me versus without me, and he chose to be with me and all of my issues. That's what love is.

Falling in love with Paul allowed me to reach a whole new level of comfort with myself and my HIV status. Growing up, I was desperately seeking normal. While I understood the reality of being HIV positive, I didn't want to have to think about it. I couldn't really talk about it anyway, most of the time, so it was easier to just tuck it away. I never really identified myself with HIV. I wanted so badly to be normal, whatever that is, that I paid as little attention to my HIV-ness as possible. I maintained a strict protocol of medication adherence and regular doctor visits, but beyond that, I kept that part of my life safely tucked under the rug. It was like the Great and Powerful Oz behind the curtain; we all know he's there, but we're really not supposed to pay attention to him. Or like Fight Club: just don't talk about it. So I was living my life keeping this very significant part of me very securely squirreled away.

When Paul and I started our life together, it was an affirmation for me that it I could live a normal life and be HIV positive—all at the same time! I could pull the curtain back. I could talk about Fight Club! Paul's unconditional love and support made me feel that even if I did encounter a negative reaction to my HIV status, I wouldn't have to face it alone. Not only did I have my family to back me up, but now I had Paul too. Someone who chose to be with me. Someone who had the option to walk away and didn't.

> *Do what you will, always*
> *Walk where you like, your steps*
> *Do as you please, I'll back you up*

Dave Matthews knows what he's talking about. I tried to get him to officiate our wedding, but as it turned out, he's quite popular and a little busy. There are always vow-renewing ceremonies, of which there will be many. Seriously, if your wedding day is supposed to be the happiest day of your life, why do it only once? Elizabeth Taylor knew what I'm talking about— although I do plan to keep the same groom for all of my upcoming nuptials. But think about it: you get to be the center of attention, drink champagne, get presents, and wear an awesome dress? Yes please! And again, in between all vow-renewals, it is perfectly acceptable to wear your wedding dress wherever and whenever you want. Seriously, I checked, it's okay.

CHAPTER FIFTEEN

"GOOD morning, Mrs. G," Paul said to me on the morning after our wedding. Music to my ears. How lucky was I to find someone to share this life with?

One of the greatest things about being married is that now there is someone to drag along to all sorts of events. As an introvert, Paul was not exactly thrilled at this prospect, but he was still a good sport. One Saturday morning in October, I dragged him out of bed at the crack of dawn to do an 8K run to benefit our pediatric cardiac program at work. We guzzled down some coffee and gathered at the starting line, trying to stay warm on the chilly fall morning. Paul started first, in the group that was actually running the 8K. I started with the second group, the group running/walking the 2K. I had no hopes of running the 8K, as my repaired heart defect put some limitations on how much physical activity I could endure. My dreams of becoming an

Olympic marathon runner had been squashed years ago, and that was fine by me. So I lined up with a bunch of moms with strollers and got ready to tackle the 2K.

Feeling robust and energetic, I started off with light jog. Oh yeah, I was trucking right along. Excuse me, jogger stroller, coming through! This is a piece of cake. I can step it up. I quickened my pace to a steady run and sailed by everyone else. It was so chilly I was anxious to get going so I could warm up. After a few more paces, my breathing started to get more shallow. The cold air bit at my lungs with each breath, and I couldn't breathe deeply enough to get a full breath. I tried to concentrate on getting a deep breath in, but it just resulted in a shallow wheeze.

Then, I started to feel the echo in my ears that made the outside world sound fuzzy and distant. I knew this feeling. This is what I felt right before I pass out. This had happened many times before, in the clinic, when I had IVs placed, or when they took large amounts of blood. It was usually a combination of low blood pressure, dehydration, some sort of painful stimuli, and my residual cardiac issues. I basically had a sensitive little heart, but I could usually predict when I was going to be in a situation where I would be prone to passing out.

This was new. I had always been able to run short distances, and this had never happened. I slowed down to a walk and tried to catch my breath. The echoing got deeper and I couldn't catch my breath, so I walked off the path to a tree and knelt down. I put my head between my knees and breathed in through my nose and out through my mouth. I could tell that someone was following me, but I couldn't see who it was because my vision went black. Then everything just turned off.

I woke up a few minutes later, still crouched down by the tree. Looking up, I saw a woman crouched next to me, rubbing my back.

"Are you okay?" she asked.

"Yeah," I replied. "I have a cardiac condition, and this happens sometimes. I've never had it happen like this though."

"You're looking a little better."

"Thank you so much for helping me. Oh my God, this is so embarrassing."

"Don't be silly. I'm just glad you're okay."

"Yeah, I'm okay. I'm feeling better."

"How about if we walk back and get you some water?"

"Okay, yeah. But you don't have to walk back. You can finish the race."

"No, I don't want you to walk back on your own. Seriously, it's okay."

We got up and started walking against the stream of the crowd.

"So has this ever happened before?" she asked.

"Well, it has, but never from running. I've passed out before when I've had a lot of blood taken, but never like this."

"You should probably get it checked out. Do you have a doctor?"

Do I ever.

"Yeah, I do. I'll call them and get it checked out."

As we continued to walk upstream, everyone looked at us as if to say, *Um, wrong way, people. Haven't you ever seen an arrow before?*

Back at the starting point, I sat down and had a banana, a granola bar, and some water and waited for Paul to cross the finish line. He rounded the bend and came over to me.

"Hey," he said, out of breath.

"Hey," I said. "How was it?"

"Good," he said. "How'd you do?"

"Well . . . I had a bit of an adventure."

"Huh?"

"Yeah, I passed out a little."

"What?!"

"Yeah. Right over there by that tree. This nice woman stayed with me and helped me back."

"Oh my God, are you okay? You've run before without passing out. Is there something wrong? We should go to the emergency room."

"No, I'm fine! I'm back to normal now. I'm just really hungry now so we should go to Bob Evans."

"Okay. Are you sure you're okay? I'm worried. How do you know if you're okay?"

"I feel much better. I'll call my doctor and see what they think."

So I learned two important things that day. One: I should have listened to my instincts that told me that waking up at 6am on a Saturday was a bad idea, for so many reasons. And two: maybe cardiac patients should be careful when running a benefit race for cardiac patients.

I called my doctor and asked for her recommendation. I had a pediatric cardiologist whom I saw for yearly check-ups, but I figured that as a 26-year-old, it might be time to start seeing an adult cardiologist. She referred me to a cardiologist within her health system.

My first visit involved the typical cardiology tests—an echocardiogram and an EKG to get a snapshot of the anatomy and functioning of my heart. They both looked good. I went home strapped to a Holter monitor, which is a portable heart monitor that stays on for 24 hours. I walked around for a day looking like the Unibomber or a police informant, all wired up.

The results of the Holter monitor were also normal. They could find nothing wrong with my heart, apart from a slight murmur that had always been there since my surgery. While good news was . . . good . . . I still wanted to find out what had happened. My family was concerned with what was happening, and I kept them updated with all my results.

"Everything was normal on the tests," I told my mom.

"I know honey, but you have to keep pressing," she said. "If we hadn't insisted on that cardiac cath when you were a toddler, they never would have found your tetrology, and you probably would have died. You have a way of fooling diagnostic tests, you little brat, so you can't let them just pass this off."

"Hey!"

"Well, it's true."

"Okay, I'll go in for a second opinion."

I made another appointment with another doctor in the practice. This one was much younger, and more aggressive with his approach. He wanted me to have an electrophysiology (EP) study to assess the electrical conductivity of my heart.

"If one of your nodes is firing wrong, that could cause serious problems, including passing out like this."

"Okay. What happens if there is something wrong with the nodes?"

"Then we would think about a pacemaker."

Seriously? I had kind of assumed that I would be done with all my cardiac drama, but apparently not. The idea of getting a pacemaker scared me, but at least he had a hunch to go on. I was glad that we were doing this test to make sure that things were really okay.

"So what does this test involve?"

"I'll give you a light sedative, and then we'll thread a catheter in through your groin up to your heart. We may put in a couple of catheters."

Cool. Why not?

"The end of that catheter will incite an electrical response in your heart — sort of zap it — and we'll be able to see how it responds. It will take about 20 minutes, then we'll have you lie flat for a few hours and then you'll go home."

"This is done awake? No anesthesia?"

"Yes, it's really not that bad. I've done hundreds of these."

Congratulations. Not that bad for you, maybe. You're the zapper, not the zappee.

"Okay, when do we schedule it?"

"As soon as possible."

My mom came down from Pennsylvania to be there with Paul and me for the procedure. We arrived at the outpatient procedure area of the hospital at six in the morning to get checked in. Paul was more in need of a sedative at that point than I was.

They called my name to go back and get ready.

"I'll be fine," I reassured him. "They'll call you back once they get me all ready."

Back in the pre-op area, I changed into a gown and the nurse started my IV. She went over my history, and asked me a few questions.

"Have you had anything to eat or drink today?" she asked.

"Nope."

"Good. How old are you?"

"Twenty-six."

"Ha. You're my youngest patient of the day by far!"
Thanks?

"Do you have any questions?"

"How sedated will I be? Will I be awake at all?"
Please say no.

"You'll be awake enough to respond to us, but you'll be so doped up that you won't really care what's happening. And you won't remember anything when we are done. Trust me, you'll be fine."

"Okay."

She didn't start any fluids through my IV; I figured that was because the procedure would be so quick they wouldn't need to do that.

Paul and my mom came back as I waited in pre-op

for my turn. We listened to the patients in the bays next to me. Not being a member of the Greatest Generation myself, I didn't really have much in common with these folks. The three of us chuckled at me being the outcast of the group.

When it was my turn, they unlocked the wheels on my stretcher and wheeled me back to the procedure room. Just before I passed through the doors, I gave Paul and my mom a kiss.

"Love you. I'll be fine," I told Paul.

"I know. I love you too."

"I'll see you when I'm done."

"Okay. Love you."

The procedure room was an octagonal room of stark white and metal.

"Hi there," the nurse said. "I'm going to be taking care of you in here."

"Hi. When do I get those sedatives?"

"Just a couple of minutes. We're going to get things ready first."

Oh good. I'll just stare at your shiny instruments until you are ready.

Several other people came in to complete their procedural duties, including my doctor.

"Hi Jamie," he said. "How are you doing?"

"Good. So I'm not going to remember any of this? And I'm not going to feel it?"

"You'll be very happy in just a few minutes."

"Okay good."

A few minutes ready, the nurse anesthetist was ready to give me my long-awaited drugs, thank God.

"You'll start to feel out of it pretty soon."

Meanwhile, the nurse started to prep the area on my groin where they were going to insert the catheters.

"Are you doing that right now? Before I'm sedated?"

"You're fine. I'm just getting things ready. I'm just going to start off with a shot of lidocaine to numb the area. Just a little pinch."

"How are you feeling?" asked the nurse anesthetist.

"Awake."

"Don't worry, you'll start to feel out of it pretty soon."

The room started to get a little hazy, but I could still hear and see everything that was going on.

"Okay, I'm going to insert the catheter now. You tell me if you can feel anything, okay?"

"Okay."

I felt pressure and pain on the insertion site. She was pushing down hard on my groin, and I felt a sharp pain with each push.

"I feel that," I said. "Can I have more medicine?"

"Okay, I can give you a little more."

"Okay. Thank you."

He pushed more drugs into my IV and I felt a little more out of it, but I could still feel everything that was happening. With the extra drugs on board at that point, it was harder for me to speak up and tell them that it was hurting.

Then I felt a pounding in my chest that I had never felt before. My heart was beating faster and harder than I had ever felt, and I thought it was going to explode.

"Something's happening," I slurred. "Something's wrong with my heart."

"That's what's supposed to happen. That's normal," the doctor said.

Well, thanks for telling me ahead of time.

"Can you give me more? I feel everything," I said.

No one answered and they kept going.

I felt a tear slide down my face and drip into my ear. The cumulative effects of the drugs did finally start to kick in, just as they were finishing up. I faded in and out of sleep as they wheeled me out into recovery to see Paul and my mom.

"Hi Sweetie," my mom said.

"Hi love," Paul said.

"I felt everything," I replied, and went back to sleep.

They took us to an inpatient room so I could fully recover and lie flat for a few hours. This was no problem, because by this time, I was completely wiped out. I slept for about five hours, waking briefly for a few minutes here and there. The nurse came in periodically to check the incision site for bleeding.

"How are you feeling?" he asked.

"Better."

"You're the youngest patient we've seen around here for a while."

"Yeah, I get that a lot."

"Well, just rest and in a few hours, we'll have you sit up and get ready to go home."

Several hours later I felt more awake, and was able to start sitting up a bit. The meal service had come by with dinner, which consisted of some sort of unidentifiable meat and something that could be either mashed potatoes or macaroni and cheese. I drank the juice, and left the rest for my 91-year-old roommate.

"All right, you want to try getting up?" the nurse asked.

"Sure."

"Okay, start slow. Just sit up on the edge of the bed for a few minutes."

I did as instructed and waited a few minutes. Then I slowly got up and my mom walked with me to the bathroom.

"You good?" she asked.

"Yup."

I closed the door to the bathroom and started to sit down. I looked at the half-used roll of toilet paper and in that instant, everything started to get dark. Two inches above the toilet paper was the nurse call button.

I should probably push that, I thought, as everything went black.

A few minutes later I still hadn't come out of the bathroom, so Paul walked towards the door. Under the door, he saw water flowing out. Panicked, he opened the door to find me wedged in between the toilet and the wall, soaked, and completely unconscious.

"GET THAT GUY!" he yelled, referring to the nurse.

The nurse ran in and scooped me up with one arm, and rushed me over to the bed.

"CALL A CODE!" the nurse yelled.

By this time, I was starting to regain consciousness. I couldn't see anything, but I heard people yelling.

"What did she have done today?"

"Get a blood glucose."

"70 over 30."

"Sugars are good."

"She's coming out of it."

I opened my eyes and saw about 15 people around me, in a frenzied state. My mom was next to me holding my hand. I looked over at her, and squeezed her hand.

"Is Paul okay?" I asked.

"Yes, he's okay. They took him out to the hall."

I nodded and saw everyone calm down and trickle out of the room as I continued to wake up. A minute later Paul slowly walked in, looking at me with wide eyes.

"Look who's back," my mom said to Paul, reassuring him that I was okay.

He walked over to the side of the bed, sat down next to me grabbed my hand, and started crying.

"It's okay. I'm fine," I said. Then I started crying, because I hated seeing him this upset.

My mom came over to comfort us both.

"She's okay. She's gotten through worse than this before," she said, as she gave Paul a hug from the side.

Paul leaned over to hug me and we took some deep breaths together.

The nurse came back after a few minutes. "How ya feeling? You gave us quite the scare."

"I know. Sorry. I'm feeling much better. I don't have to stay overnight now do I?"

"Well, after that little stunt, I'm not sure. We'll see

how things go. You should get something to eat."

"Yes," my mom said, "I'm going to the cafeteria and I'll get you some real food. What do you want?"

"Anything."

"Got it."

She came back with a tray piled high with pizza, French fries, juice, pudding, salad, fruit, a brownie, and a few other things. I ate nearly all of it. This day of no eating or drinking, no IV fluids, a painful procedure, and nearly dying left me quite famished.

It was just what I needed. My second attempt at getting up was exceedingly more successful than the first. The doctor came in to watch me walk down the hall and back. Having accomplished this task, I was given my walking papers and released. I got dressed and walked out of the room, past my little old roommate.

"Sorry for the excitement," I said as I walked by.

"Meh," she replied, unimpressed.

The outcome of that whole ordeal yielded normal test results. All of that, and we still didn't have any information. I was thankful that I didn't have to have a pacemaker, but still concerned that something was wrong. I was still feeling dizzier and nearly passing out more often than usual.

I found a third cardiologist who specialized in adults with congenital heart defects like me. Ding ding! I found a winner. I came to him with all of my issues and he had me go through a few more tests—nothing at all invasive or exciting as the EP study. He advised me to increase my fluids and cut back on my caffeine intake, which happened to be that of a cross-country trucker.

Doing this helped greatly, and my symptoms started to subside. Time to get back to the newlywed thing. This little cardiac hiccup took us both by surprise, since my issue du jour had been HIV for the longest time. Poor Paul. I had put him through enough for an entire lifetime and we hadn't even been married for a year. We were quite ready for things to get back to normal.

CHAPTER SIXTEEN

LOOKING back at my winding road of growing up with HIV, I realize how much I have learned and how much the future excites me. My life has taught me to step forward positively (yes, irony is fun, isn't it?) and to appreciate everything. Okay, almost everything; it is very hard to appreciate some things, like cavities or people who write checks at the grocery store.

It would be very cheesy of me to say that every day is a gift, so I won't. There are certainly days that have not been gifts. Or if they are, then they're sick, twisted gifts. But remember what my mom says: "This too shall pass." Those non-gift days will eventually make way for better days to come. That's what keeps me going. Even if that's a very idealistic, My Little Pony way of seeing the world, that's fine by me. I love ponies.

I've always believed that if you have something to

look forward to, it keeps you going when times are tough. This is how I see birthdays. Each birthday is a goal that I look forward to with great anticipation. When I hear people lamenting about an upcoming milestone birthday, I can't relate. I honestly want to smack them. To me, birthdays are events to celebrate and appreciate wholeheartedly.

When I learned about my HIV status as a little kid, I didn't know if I had a future, and if I did, what it would hold for me. When I was 10, I wanted so badly to turn 20, not only because I wanted to survive that long, but because I just thought 20 was a really cool age. During those first years of my treatment and drug protocols, my prognosis got better by the day, and I began to see hope on the horizon. I went from wishing and hoping that I make it to 20, to being quite certain that I would. By the time I finally did hit that milestone, I was happy and healthy and turned my focus to more milestones on the horizon. It was exhilarating! Twenty-five was a similarly exciting event. Fifteen years prior, we didn't know if I'd make it through high school, and here I was, a college graduate, establishing my career, happily married, and feeling better than ever. It was again a time to celebrate!

As I approached 30, I felt like a kid in the parking lot of an amusement park. I couldn't wait to get out of the car and soak in the excitement! I was genuinely antsy for months. It was such an amazing feeling to be doing this well, and seeing no end in sight to the milestones. It was cause for celebration — which we do very well, I might add. When you think of a 30-year-old's birthday party, you think of ponies and princess tiaras, right? Well, that's exactly how we celebrated. You see, just like every other little girl, when people ask me what I want for my birthday, Christmas, Flag Day, I reply, "A pony." This has been my answer for years. I'm not sure why people bother to ask anymore, to be perfectly honest. Well, it turns out that 30 is the lucky number for that wish!

Paul and my family planned a fantastic party at my mom's house in Gettysburg with close friends and family. We had been planning for months. On the day of the event, Paul and I drove up to my mom's house to get ready. Shortly after we arrived, a horse trailer pulled up in my mom's driveway. At first I thought that they were lost. It happens. The house was in the woods, down a long gravel driveway. From the road, it could be anything — a campsite, an Indian burial ground, a horse farm, an Ikea — anything. We often got misguided visitors whom we kindly point in the right direction (after we make sure that they are not lunatics on the loose looking for people to kidnap, of course). Once I realized that this horse-mobile was not lost, but was in fact, a surprise for my birthday, I nearly peed in my pants. (Seriously, I had consumed a lot of Diet Coke that day, and I didn't go to the bathroom before I went outside.)

So I spent a wonderful day riding my birthday horse (ours for the day, not for good), hanging out with my friends and family, and eating the best chocolate cake in the world. It couldn't have been better! Oh, and the tiara? Yes, there was one of those too. Look, they were lucky that I didn't wear my wedding dress along with the tiara.

That birthday was a precursor to many more to come. Parties, horses, you have to do it up and have fun! Note to loved ones: each birthday that ends in a zero or a five should involve a horse and diamonds. Just saying . . .

People have asked me if I ever thought about what it would be like if I didn't have HIV. Of course I have. I would have loved to not get poked and not take meds that made me sick. It would have been much less stressful not to have to hide behind the truth and lie to my friends in school. It would have been wonderful not to have to have THE TALK with every serious boyfriend. It would have been amazing not to lose friends way too soon. No one would choose to go through this pain. But fantasizing about my life without HIV is futile. No one can turn back time and change what happened on that fateful day of my surgery. This is the life that I've been given, and when I look back on the three decades that I've lived so far, the beautiful and joyous moments far outweigh the pain and heartache. Living with HIV has opened up a world of extraordinary people and experiences to me. Each and every one of those experiences has made me the person I am today. Through the dark came an infinitely brighter light.

I know full well that I can only feel this way because I have been so incredibly lucky. I recovered well from my cardiac problems. I received HIV medications just in the nick of time. I had a supportive family carry me every step of the way. I found a match in Paul, who lovingly and willingly accepts me and all that my life brings with it.

I know that this doesn't happen for everyone. I've seen friends whose families couldn't take care of them the way mine took care of me. I've seen people try and fail on so many medications. I've seen the pain of this disease turn people to addiction. I've seen stigma and hatred that other people have had to endure. I've seen people give up.

I thank my lucky stars every day that I have been so fortunate. Life has put a lot of challenges in my path, but it's also given me the tools to get through those challenges. Instead of leaving me wounded, it left me stronger.

I've come to place now where I have a normal life expectancy. Paul and I can look forward to a full life together. If we choose to, we could have our own child with a 98-99% chance our baby would be born without HIV. If my meds fail, I have a variety of others to try. These realities did not exist for me 20, or even 10 years ago. Options were non-existent at the beginning, when crossing my fingers was often my best option.

Now, I can look back at my journey thus far and know that it's nowhere near finished. There are countless more adventures to come. There will undoubtedly be more roadblocks along the way. My life has never followed a normal path, and I don't expect that to change. Luckily, my abnormal path has brought more joy than pain, and has given me so much more than it has taken. I've already packed a lifetime of experiences into my 33 years. And the best is yet to come.

ACKNOWLEDGEMENTS

This book—and my very existence—wouldn't be possible without the people in my life. My family got me through the most critical times of my life with hope and love. Heather and Kelly, you often had to take a backseat to my medical drama, and you did it with grace and love. Through it all—even the tough stuff— you were there to have fun with me and take care of me. Even though I'll never admit it, I know I was a spoiled little punk sometimes and I'm thankful that you put up with me. I'm so lucky to be your little sister.

Dad, you would go to the ends of the earth for me, and I have felt that every day of my life. You have taught me so much about what it means to work hard and enjoy life at the same time. I hope I have made you proud. I'm forever grateful for your support and encouragement as I have written this book. Your unconditional love and support means the world to me. Words can't describe how lucky I feel to have you as my dad.

Mom, you have always been my partner in crime and I cherish the bond that we have. You were with me every step of the way, as my number one advocate and nurturer. The times that we spent together in clinics and hospitals are some of the most cherished moments of my life. You got me through all of the tough stuff and taught me how to cope and carry on with hope. I wouldn't be the person I am today without you. You mean more to me than you will ever know. I wish everyone could have a mom like you.

Paul, Edie, and Julie, thank you for your encouragement and love. You welcomed me into your lives with open arms and I feel lucky to have you as my extended family. I love you all.

My wonderful editor Dr. Lori Handelman, you helped me bring this book from an ambitious idea to a finished product that I can hold with pride. Thank you for your honestly, your expertise, and your counsel. I hope that this is the first of many projects together.

I have been blessed with amazing friends my entire life. To my Hole in the Wall family, Gettysburg HS friends, Penn State beauties, Child Life girls, and many others: thank you for unending support and laughter. You have filled up my soul and I love you all for it.

Cami Frickman, thank you for giving me the gift of your artistic talent for my book cover. It means so much to me that you were a part of this. You are one of the most genuine people that I know, and your love and support have meant so much to me. I'm so glad that I always have a friend with me in Inappropriate-ville. Love you.

Paul, you gave me the strength and self-confidence to open up about my life and write this book. Your love is unconditional and it builds me up every day. I know that no matter what happens, you will be there with me. You are so good to me and I can't believe I get to be married to you. You're my best friend on the planet and I love you big time.

In gratitude and love...

ABOUT THE AUTHOR

Wait, isn't this whole book about the author? Jamie earned a BS in Biobehavioral Health from Penn State University and a Masters in Public Health from Walden University. She completed her child life internship at Children's Hospital at Dartmouth, and has been in the child life profession for over ten years. She lives in Northern Virginia with her husband of seven years and beloved dog Lucy.

Jamie is an experienced public speaker. She appeared on the Oprah Winfrey Show in 1997 for a World AIDS Day special. Jamie has also spoken at the annual Elizabeth Glaser Pediatric AIDS Foundation A Time for Heroes event in Los Angeles. She has also addressed post-doctoral students at the National Institutes of Health and Georgetown Medical School students. As an Ambassador for the Elizabeth Glaser Pediatric AIDS Foundation, she has also spoken at a Town Hall meeting for President Obama's National HIV/AIDS agenda planning. She was also a featured speaker at an event sponsored by the United Nations Association of the National Capital Area, the US Agency for International Development (USAID), and Maternal and Child Health Integrated Programs (MCHIP). Most recently, Jamie was a keynote speaker and group facilitator at the 19th Annual International AIDS Conference in Washington DC.

Jamie is passionate about health education and advocating for the rights of children and families undergoing medical experiences, and continuing the fight to eliminate AIDS.

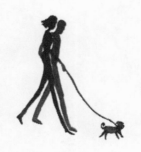

17956741R00142

Made in the USA
Charleston, SC
08 March 2013